全国高等学校教材
供临床、预防、基础、口腔、药学、护理等专业用

教师
用书

医学专业英语
阅读二分册

总主编　白永权

主　编　卢凤香

副主编　吴　青

编　委　（按姓氏笔画排序）

王梦杰　西安交通大学

卢凤香　首都医科大学

白永权　西安交通大学

任　雁　首都医科大学

华　瑶　首都医科大学

杨　波　首都医科大学

吴　青　北京中医药大学

郑艳华　西安交通大学

谢春晖　首都医科大学

人民卫生出版社

·北京·

图书在版编目（CIP）数据

医学专业英语. 阅读二分册. 教师用书/卢凤香主编. —北京：人民卫生出版社，2021.12

ISBN 978-7-117-32468-7

Ⅰ. ①医… Ⅱ. ①卢… Ⅲ. ①医学－英语－阅读教学－医学院校－教材 Ⅳ. ①R

中国版本图书馆 CIP 数据核字（2021）第 237662 号

人卫智网	www.ipmph.com	医学教育、学术、考试、健康，购书智慧智能综合服务平台
人卫官网	www.pmph.com	人卫官方资讯发布平台

医学专业英语　阅读二分册　教师用书

Yixue Zhuanye Yingyu Yuedu Er Fence Jiaoshi Yongshu

主　　编：卢凤香
出版发行：人民卫生出版社（中继线 010-59780011）
地　　址：北京市朝阳区潘家园南里 19 号
邮　　编：100021
E - mail：pmph @ pmph.com
购书热线：010-59787592　010-59787584　010-65264830
印　　刷：河北新华第一印刷有限责任公司
经　　销：新华书店
开　　本：787 × 1092　1/16　　**印张：**5
字　　数：122 千字
版　　次：2021 年 12 月第 1 版
印　　次：2022 年 1 月第 1 次印刷
标准书号：ISBN 978-7-117-32468-7
定　　价：30.00 元

打击盗版举报电话：010-59787491　E-mail：WQ @ pmph.com
质量问题联系电话：010-59787234　E-mail：zhiliang @ pmph.com

修订说明

《医学专业英语》系列教材自 2001 年出版以来，深受广大医学英语教师、医学生和医务工作者的欢迎，许多医学院校一直在使用，先后印刷二十多次。我国香港特别行政区和国外一些医学院校也以不同的方式选用了该套教材。2016 年人民卫生出版社决定对这套教材进行修订，我们再次组织全国医学院校中精通医学英语教学和教材编写的老师，包括部分参加过编写第 1 版教材的老师，在保留原有教材实用、专业和规范的特点和风格同时，对该套教材进行了一次认真、全面的修改，使之更贴近医学生的学习需求，更好地满足我国医学英语教学的需要，进一步体现教材服务于医学教育和追踪医学科学发展前沿的本质，切实提高医学生的医学英语应用能力。

本次修订的重点是对全套教材进行重新梳理，改正第 1 版教材中的疏漏之处；适当降低全套教材的难度；适度压缩各分册的内容；调整某些章节的先后顺序；删除教学效果不佳和不符合当前教学实际要求的课文和练习；换入一批可读性更强、体现医学科学最新知识的文章和更能培养学生英语语言输出能力的练习。

本次修订的原则如下。

1. 本套教材的修订以《大学英语教学指南》为指导，依据当代专门用途英语教学理念，引用网络和多媒体等现代教育技术，进行修订和编写。本套教材的原有定位不变，以我国大学英语四级水平为起点，供临床、预防、基础、口腔、药学和护理等专业的本科生和硕士研究生学习使用。

2. 修订后本套教材共六册，其中学生用书三册：《医学专业英语　阅读一分册》《医学专业英语　阅读二分册》（合称《阅读分册》）和《医学专业英语　听说分册》（简称《听说分册》）；教师用书三册：《医学专业英语　阅读一分册教师用书》《医学专业英语　阅读二分册教师用书》和《医学专业英语　听说分册教师用书》。

3. 阅读、听说两种教材都独立自成体系，但又相互关联形成一个整体。在教学中每种教材既可单独使用，也可根据实际需要将两种教材组合在一起使用。每册教材可满足 40 学时的课内教学使用，全套教材可供 120 学时的教学使用。

4. 《阅读分册》与《听说分册》每章的主题基本相同，都是同一个医学人体系统。在编写英语系列教材时，采用每册中每章主题相同的编写模式既是对英语教材编写体例的创新，也更适合医学英语教学。学生从阅读和听说不同角度学习同一个医学人体系统的常用医学英语术语构词形式和该系统人体结构、生理和常见疾病的英语词汇和英语表述。

医学英语是很多国家和地区的医学生都要学习的一门课程，差异只是学时的多少和内容的深浅。母语是英语的医学生只学习医学英语词汇学，而母语是非英语的医学生需要将普通英语和医学英语结合起来,起点低而且学时多。在本套教材的修订和编写过程中,我们充分考虑到了我国医学英语教育的现状以及医学生学习医学英语的实际需要和存在的难点,力争编写出一套适合我国医学英语教学的优秀医学英语教材。

本次修订中,各位编者认真负责,对每个分册都进行了大幅度的调整和改编。新版《听说分册》增加了大量新音频,使得语料更加真实活泼;《阅读分册》新选了许多可读性更强的文章,同时对原书每篇文章的长度都做了适当压缩。在练习的配置方面,更加突出了对医学生英语语言输出能力的培养,增加了大量说、写和译的练习。

《医学专业英语》系列教材第1版和第2版都由白永权教授担任总主编。第1版的《医学专业英语 阅读一分册》由邱望生担任主编,郝长江担任副主编,编者有陈忠荣、张帆和郝军;《医学专业英语 阅读二分册》由张宏清担任主编,周铁成担任副主编,编者有胡建、葛广纯、王群英和孙秋丹;《医学专业英语 听说分册》由董双辰担任主编,梁平担任副主编,编者有王文秀、陈春林和潘宏声。第2版的《医学专业英语 阅读一分册》由范晓晖担任主编,李永安、熊淋宵担任副主编,编者有朱元、王丹、李权芳、易超、穆文超、晏国莉和张鹏;《医学专业英语 阅读二分册》由卢凤香担任主编,吴青担任副主编,编者有谢春晖、任雁、华瑶、杨波、王梦杰和郑艳华;《医学专业英语 听说分册》及教师用书由陈向京担任主编,孙庆祥担任副主编,编者有李莹、晏国莉、戴月珍、凌秋虹、詹菊红和陈英。

参加《医学专业英语》系列教材两版编写的院校有西安交通大学、北京大学、复旦大学、首都医科大学、北京中医药大学、青岛大学、陕西中医药大学、四川大学、华中科技大学、中南大学、吉林大学、中山大学、南方医科大学、海军军医大学(原第二军医大学)、陆军军医大学(原第三军医大学)、空军军医大学(原第四军医大学)、哈尔滨医科大学、河北医科大学、山东大学、兰州大学和承德医学院。

本次修订过程中,许多教授、学者和领导付出了很大心血,在此对他们表示衷心的感谢。

《医学专业英语》系列教材出版以来,我们收集到了一些宝贵意见和建议,这为我们做好第2版的修订工作提供了十分宝贵和可靠的依据和资料。在此谨向提出意见和建议的各位读者,向所有使用这套教材的老师和同学,表示深深的敬意和感谢,欢迎你们今后一如既往地不吝指教。

白永权

2021 年 11 月

前　言

　　本书为《医学专业英语》系列教材的阅读第二分册，以我国大学英语四级水平为起点，供临床、预防、基础、口腔、药学和护理等专业的本科生和硕士研究生学习医学专业英语使用。

　　编写宗旨

　　《医学专业英语　阅读二分册》旨在帮助学生学习人体解剖系统的医学英语术语以及人体各系统结构、生理和常见疾病的英语词汇和英语表达，通过听、说、读、写、译多方面进行医学英语语言知识的操练，培养学生的医学英语语言表达能力和综合应用能力。

　　全书框架

　　本册共 9 章，眼与耳、内分泌系统、泌尿系统、生殖系统、神经系统、皮肤、肿瘤学、药物以及医学高科技。每章都包括医学词汇（Medical Terminology）和阅读短文（Reading Passages）两大部分。

　　Section A　Medical Terminology

　　医学词汇部分每章都讲授 20 个左右本系统常用的构词形式和前后缀，并配有 3 类有利于医学词汇学习和记忆的练习。

　　Section B　Reading Passages

　　阅读部分每章都包括 3 篇有关人体同一系统或同一主题的文章，除了第一、二和九章外，每章的主题都是一个系统，学生将学习该系统的常用医学英语术语构词形式和该系统人体结构、生理功能和常见疾病的英语词汇和英语表达。第 1 篇是关于该系统解剖和生理功能的短文；第 2 篇是有关该系统病理和疾病的概述；第 3 篇是该系统的某个特定疾病。3 篇文章的内容由浅入深、相互呼应，难度和长度逐篇加大。

　　第 1 篇和第 2 篇文章后各配四类练习。每个练习都有明确的目的。

● 配对和句子填空类练习考查学生对本课基本词汇和主要知识的掌握。

● 段落填空类练习进一步训练学生的语句表达技能，强调语句内在的逻辑关系和语义关联。

● 短语、句子和段落的汉英及英汉翻译类练习培养学生的语言综合应用能力。

● 任务型口头回答问题类练习培养学生学以致用的口语表达能力。

　　第 3 篇文章后配有两类练习。

● 判断正误或多项选择类练习考查学生对课文主旨大意和重要细节的理解。

● 医学词汇构成分析类练习进一步培养学生运用构词法知识辨识单词意思的能力。

　　为了便于读者学习和查阅生词，在本书的后面附有总词汇表。

本册阅读可供 40 个学时的教学使用。在具体使用时，根据学生的英语水平和课程时数决定是全部使用，还是选用某一部分或某几篇文章。一般来说，词汇部分是必学的，阅读部分的 3 篇文章可根据学生的不同水平来选用，剩余的文章留给学有余力的学生自学。

修订特色

结合我国医学英语教育的现状以及医学生学习医学英语的实际需要，在保持第 1 版原有定位和特色的前提下，本册教材修订的总体目标是使本教材更贴近医学英语教学的实际需要和学生的实际水平。修订的重点是适当降低难度和更换教学效果不佳或不太符合当前教学实际的课文和练习。为此，我们对本书主要做了以下两方面的修订：

➤ 更换了原书近三分之一的文章，删除了原书中内容过时或过于专业、语言难度过大的文章，新选了一批可读性更强、更具时代感的文章。

➤ 对所有练习的形式和内容进行了必要的修改，对原有的练习重新排序，使其更符合由易到难循序渐进的学习原则。

本书由卢凤香担任主编，吴青担任副主编，谢春晖、任雁、华瑶、杨波、王梦杰和郑艳华参与编写。

由于时间紧迫和编者水平有限，书中难免会存在缺点和错误，望同行和读者不吝赐教。

编　者

2021 年 11 月

Contents

Chapter One Eyes and Ears

 Section A   Medical Terminology

Learn the following combining forms, prefixes and suffixes for the eyes and ears and try to write in the blank space the literal meaning both in English and Chinese of the provided terminology.

Word Part	Meaning	Example Term	Meaning in English and Chinese
acous/o	sound 声音；hearing 听觉	acoustic /ə'kuːstɪk/	pertaining to sound or hearing 声音的, 听觉的
		acoustics /ə'kuːstɪks/	study of sound 声学
audi/o	hearing 听	audiology /ˌɔːdɪ'ɒlədʒɪ/	study of hearing disorders 听觉学
		audiometry /ˌɔːdɪ'ɒmətrɪ/	measurement of hearing 测听术
audit/o	hearing 听	auditory /'ɔːdɪtərɪ/	pertaining to the sense of hearing 听觉的
		audition /ɔː'dɪʃən/	capability of hearing 听力
aur/o	external ear (外)耳	aural /'ɔːrəl/	pertaining to the ear or hearing 耳的, 听觉的
		aurinasal /ˌɔːrɪ'neɪsl/	pertaining to the ear and nose 耳鼻的
blephar/o	eyelid 眼睑	blepharedema /ˌblefərɪ'diːmə/	swelling of the eyelid 眼睑水肿
		blepharitis /blefə'raɪtɪs/	inflammation of the eyelid 眼睑炎
choroid/o	choroids 脉络膜	choroiditis /ˌkɔːrɔɪ'daɪtɪs/	inflammation of the choroid 脉络膜炎
		choroidectomy /ˌkɔːrɔɪ'dektəmɪ/	surgical removal of the choroid 脉络膜切除术
cili/o	ciliary 睫状的	cilioretinal /ˌsɪlɪə'retɪnəl/	pertaining to the ciliary body and the retina 睫状体视网膜的
		ciliospinal /ˌsɪlɪə'spaɪnəl/	pertaining to the ciliary body and the spine 睫状体脊髓的
corne/o	cornea 角膜	corneitis /ˌkɔːnɪ'aɪtɪs/	inflammation of the cornea 角膜炎
		corneocyte /'kɔːniːəʊˌsaɪt/	cells having the feature of cornea 角层细胞
-(a)cusis	hearing 听觉	anacusis /ənə'kjuːsɪs/	without sense of hearing 聋
		presbycusis /ˌprezbɪ'kjuːsɪs/	deafness that occurs with the process of aging 老年性耳聋

Continue

Word Part	Meaning	Example Term	Meaning in English and Chinese
dacry/o	tear duct 泪管	dacryorrhea /ˌdækriːəˈrɪə/	overflow of tears 流泪
		dacryostenosis /ˌdækriːɒstəˈnəʊsɪs/	constriction of a tear duct 泪管狭窄
ir/o	iris 虹膜	iritis /aɪəˈraɪtɪs/	inflammation of the iris 虹膜炎
		iritomy /ɪˈrɪtəmɪ/	surgical incision of the iris 虹膜切开术
labyrinth/o	labyrinth 内耳迷路	labyrinthitis /ˌlæbərɪnˈθaɪtɪs/	inflammation of the labyrinth 内耳迷路炎
		labyrinthotomy /ˌlæbərɪnˈθɔːtəmɪ/	incision of the labyrinth 迷路切开术
lacrim/o	tears 泪	lacrimal /ˈlækrɪml/	pertaining to tears 泪腺的
		lacrimator /ˈlækrəˌmeɪtə/	tear promoting agent 催泪剂
ocul/o, ophthalm/o	eye 眼	oculist /ˈɒkjʊlɪst/	physician specialized in the eyes 眼科医生
		intraocular /ˌɪntrəˈɒkjʊlə/	inside of the eyes 眼内的
		ophthalmology /ˌɒfθælˈmɒlədʒɪ/	study of the eyes 眼科学
		exophthalmos /ˌeksɒfˈθælməs/	protrusion of the eyeball 眼球突出症
-opia	eye 眼；vision 视力	hemianopia /ˌhemɪəˈnəʊpɪə/	blindness in one half of the visual field 偏盲
		hyperopia /ˌhaɪpəˈrəʊpɪə/	farsightedness 远视
opt/o	vision 视力；eye 眼	optometer /ɒpˈtɒmɪtə/	an instrument measuring vision 视力计
		optometry /ɒpˈtɒmətrɪ/	measurement of the eyes and vision 验光
ot/o	ear 耳	otoscopy /əʊˈtɒskəpɪ/	visual examination of the ear 耳镜检查
		otorhinology /ˌɒtəʊraɪˈnɒlədʒɪ/	study of the ear and the nose 耳鼻科学
pupill/o	pupil 瞳孔	pupillary /ˈpjuːpɪlərɪ/	pertaining to the pupil 瞳孔的
		pupilloscope /ˈpjuːpɪləˌskəʊp/	instrument for examining the pupils 瞳孔镜
retin/o	retina 视网膜	retinopathy /retɪˈnɒpəθɪ/	disease of the retina 视网膜病
		retinitis /ˌretɪˈnaɪtɪs/	inflammation of the retina 视网膜炎
scler/o	sclera 巩膜	scleritis /skləˈraɪtɪs/	inflammation of the sclera 巩膜炎
		episclera /ˌepɪskˈlɪərə/	outermost layer of the sclera 巩膜外层
tympan/o	eardrum 鼓室；鼓膜	tympanic /tɪmˈpænɪk/	pertaining to the eardrum 鼓室的，鼓膜的
		tympanoplasty /ˌtɪmpænəʊˈplæstɪ/	surgical repair of the eardrum 鼓膜成形术
vestibul/o	vestibule 前庭	vestibulotomy /ˌvestɪbjʊˈlɒtəmɪ/	incision into the vestibule 前庭切开术
		vestibulitis /ˌvestɪbjʊˈlaɪtɪz/	inflammation of the vestibule 前庭炎

Exercises

Ⅰ. Write the definitions of the following combining forms and provide an example word for each of them.

		Definition	Medical Term
1.	-cusis	hearing	presbycusis
2.	corne/o	cornea	corneitis
3.	dacry/o	tear duct	dacryoma
4.	ophthalm/o	eye	ophthalmology
5.	-opia	eye, vision	hyperopia
6.	scler/o	sclera	episclera
7.	ocul/o	eye	oculopathy
8.	vestibul/o	vestibule	vestibulotomy

Ⅱ. Write a word for each of the following definitions.

1.	caused by hearing, especially a loud sound	audiogenic
2.	a device used to measure hearing	audiometer
3.	pertaining to cornea	corneal
4.	disease of the retina	retinopathy
5.	an instrument to record the responses of the pupil	pupillograph
6.	surgical repair of the ear	otoplasty
7.	inflammation of the sclera	scleritis
8.	inflammation of the iris	iritis
9.	relating to the eye or vision	optical
10.	pertaining to the lacrimal sac and nose	lacrimonasal

Ⅲ. Match each word part in Column A with its English term in Column B. Write the corresponding letter in the blank provided.

Column A		Column B
D	1. pupill/o	A. iris
E	2. cili/o	B. eye, vision
A	3. ir/o	C. sound, hearing
B	4. opt/o	D. pupil
C	5. acous/o	E. ciliary body
H	6. choroid/o	F. tear
I	7. ophthalm/o	G. eyelid
G	8. blephar/o	H. choroids
F	9. lacrim/o	I. eye
J	10. ot/o	J. ear

→ Section B Reading Passages

Passage One Eyes and Ears

Exercises

Ⅰ. Fill in the following blanks with the terms in the box.

labyrinth	lacrimal
transparency	trauma
pigmentation	irritate
dilate	lubrication

1. Cataract is a condition that affects the <u>transparency</u> of the lenses.
2. An abnormal sensitivity to light may be caused by eye inflammation, lack of <u>pigmentation</u> in the iris, or various diseases.
3. In darker surroundings, the pupils <u>dilate</u> naturally to let in more light.
4. Blunt <u>trauma</u> to the eye can create swelling and inflammation in the front half of the eye.
5. When chopped, onions contain certain chemical substances which <u>irritate</u> the eyes.
6. The <u>lacrimal</u> gland continually secretes tears to moisten and protect the surface of the eye.
7. Doctors recommend using eye drops for <u>lubrication</u> and taking a break every 15 minutes to look into the distance.
8. In most mammals, together with the cochlea, the vestibular system constitutes the <u>labyrinth</u> of the inner ear.

Ⅱ. Fill in each blank with a proper word or words.

The human visual system is designed to give us depth perception, which means that we can tell which objects are in front of or behind other objects. (1) <u>Depth perception</u> is useful for doing simple tasks, such as pouring a cup of coffee or (2) <u>driving</u> a car, and is even more important in tasks that require detailed eye-hand coordination, such as performing surgery.

How exactly are the eyes designed to give us depth perception? First, both (3) <u>eyes</u> must have normal or near normal vision to work together. (4) <u>Glasses</u> or contact lenses may be needed to obtain normal (5) <u>vision</u>. Then, the eyes must be aligned in the skull so that they are facing in the same direction and are close enough together that each eye's peripheral vision or (6) <u>side vision</u> overlaps considerably with that of the other. If we cover one eye and then the other when looking at an (7) <u>object</u>, we can tell that each eye is seeing the same object just a little (8) <u>differently</u>. As we cover and uncover each eye, it is as if each object (9) <u>moves</u> a little to the right or to the left. Therefore, each eye receives a slightly different (10) <u>image</u> that is sent to the brain for processing.

The ability of the brain to process or blend these two similar images is called fusion. The brain must be able to maintain the blending of these images into one image as the eyes move together in various directions. High-level fusion develops completely during childhood, usually between the ages of 5 and 9.

Ⅲ.Translate the following anatomical words for the ears and the eyes into English.

1. 角膜   cornea
2. 脉络膜   choroid
3. 视网膜   retina
4. 耳郭   auricle
5. 耳蜗   cochlea
6. （内耳）迷路   labyrinth
7. 鼓膜   tympanic membrane
8. 锤骨   malleus
9. 砧骨   incus
10.镫骨   stapes

Ⅳ.Answer the following questions.

1. What prevents the eye from injury?

   The sclera, the cornea, as well as eyelids and eyelashes work together to prevent the eye from injury. The sclera forms a tough outer surface that protects the inner structures of the eye, and the cornea protects the front portion of the eye.

2. What determines the eye color?

   The pigmentation of the iris determines the eye color.

3. What is the function of vitreous humor?

   In addition to its refractory function, the vitreous humor maintains pressure within the eyeball, preventing it from collapsing inward.

4. What part in the ear is responsible for balance and motion?

   The vestibules of the ear are responsible for balance and motion.

Passage Two   I am Eye

Exercises

Ⅰ. Match the terms in Column A for the diseases related to the eyes with the definitions in Column B.

Column A		Column B
C	1. blepharitis	A. paralysis of the iris
F	2. conjunctivitis	B. inflammation of the retina due to exposure to intense light
D	3. corneoiritis	C. inflammation of the eyelids
A	4. iridoplegia	D. inflammation of the cornea and the iris
G	5. iritis	E. paralysis of the eye

___B___ 6. photoretinitis   F. inflammation of the conjunctiva

___E___ 7. ophthalmoplegia   G. inflammation of the iris

Ⅱ. Translate the following eye problems and diseases into English. If necessary, you may consult a dictionary.

1. 近视眼   <u>myopia</u>
2. 散光   <u>astigmatism</u>
3. 结膜炎   <u>conjunctivitis</u>
4. 白内障   <u>cataract</u>
5. 斜视   <u>strabismus</u>
6. 飞蚊症   <u>eye floaters</u>
7. 眼干燥症   <u>dry eyes</u>
8. 青光眼   <u>glaucoma</u>
9. 夜盲症   <u>night blindness</u>
10. 色盲   <u>color blindness</u>

Ⅲ. Translate the following sentences into English.

1. 每个物体都会反光。人眼仅能感知一小部分的光，这被称为可见光谱。

   Every object reflects light. The human eye is only able to pick up on a small range of this light, called visible spectrum.

2. 遗传性眼部疾病使人们不能分辨颜色，通常被称为色盲。最常见的色盲是无法分辨红色和绿色。

   Inherited eye disorders cause people to confuse one color for another — a condition commonly called color blindness. The most common type of color blindness is the inability to distinguish red from green.

3. 光线强烈时，瞳孔几乎是关闭的；在黑暗的夜晚，瞳孔是完全张开的。

   In bright sun the pupil is nearly closed; on a dark night it is wide open.

4. 人刚出生时，视力和现在不同。刚出生时，人只能看到光和影。

   A man wasn't born with the eyes he has today. At birth, he could see only light and shadow.

5. 儿童在暗淡光线下比成人看得清楚，即使在非常不利的环境下看东西眼睛也不会受损。

   The young see better in dim light than adults; and viewing under even the most adverse circumstances does no harm.

Ⅳ. Discuss the following topics.

1. Young people today easily become near-sighted. What causes this condition? What are the effective ways to protect their eyes from becoming near-sighted?

   The answer is open.

2. What are the distinct features of eyes in the first few months of an infant?

   In the first few months, an infant is long-sighted and he can move in exact unison.

3. What common eye disorders are talked about in the passage?

   The common eye disorders discussed in the passage are glaucoma, astigmatism and cataract.

Passage Three   Lifestyle Choices and Glaucoma

Exercises

Ⅰ. Read the following statements and decide whether they are true or false. Then write T for true and F for false in the brackets.

[F] 1. According to one research on non-smoking and healthy people, aerobic exercise decreased heart rate and systolic blood pressure while increasing IOP and diastolic blood pressure.

[T] 2. Isometric and isokinetic exercises can lower IOP and its effects are proportional to exercise intensity.

[T] 3. Smoking has been associated with IOP elevation, macular degeneration and cataract.

[F] 4. According to one study IOP elevation is not proportional to musicians' force of blowing when they play high-resistance wind instruments.

[T] 5. Ginkgo biloba improves short-term visual field in patients with normal-tension glaucoma.

[F] 6. Coffee consumption increases little risk to the patients with open-angle glaucoma.

[T] 7. Excessive coffee consumption has a positive association with increased risks of glaucoma.

[F] 8. People consuming alcohol excessively stop drinking, which will lower the eye pressure suddenly.

[T] 9. Migraine and sleep apnea are linked to increased risk of glaucoma development and progression.

[T] 10. Marijuana is not recommended to treat glaucoma due to its side effects.

Ⅱ. Here is a list of terms from the text. Analyze their meanings using the word building knowledge you have learned. Leave the space empty if the word part does not apply.

Term	Prefix	Root	Suffix	Chinese Translation
1. pathogenesis		path/o-	-genesis	发病机制
2. neuropathy		neur/o-	-pathy	神经病变
3. intraocular	intra-	ocul/o-	-ar	眼内的
4. antihypertensive	anti-hyper-	tens/	-ive	抗高血压的
5. hypotensive	hypo-	tens/	-ive	低血压的
6. polyphenolic	poly-	phenol/	-ic	多酚的

Chapter Two Endocrine System

Section A   Medical Terminology

Learn the following combining forms, prefixes and suffixes for the endocrine system and try to write in the blank space the literal meaning both in English and Chinese of the provided terminology.

Word Part	Meaning	Example Term	Meaning in English and Chinese
aden/o	gland 腺	adenitis /ˌædəˈnaɪtɪs/	inflammation of a gland 腺炎
		adenopathy /ˌædɪˈnɒpəθɪ/	disease of a gland 腺病
andr/o	male 男性，雄性	androgen /ˈændrədʒən/	any substance that promotes male characteristics 雄性激素
		andrology /ænˈdrɒləʒɪ/	study of the diseases in male reproductive system 男科学
adren/o	adrenal gland 肾上腺	adrenolytic /əˌdriːnəˈlɪtɪk/	inhibiting the action of epinephrine 抗肾上腺素的
		adrenopathy /ədrɪˈnɒpəθɪ/	disease of adrenal gland 肾上腺病
calc/i	calcium 钙	calcipenia /kælsɪˈpiːnɪə/	deficiency of calcium 钙缺乏
		calciuria /kælsɪˈjuərɪə/	presence of calcium in urine 钙尿
cortic/o	cortex 皮层	corticosteroid /ˌkɔːtɪkəʊˈsterɔɪd/	any steroid hormone synthesized by the adrenal cortex 皮质类固醇
		corticoadrenal /kɔːtɪkəʊəˈdrenl/	pertaining to the cortex of the adrenal gland 肾上腺皮质的
crin/o	secretion 分泌	endocrinology /ˌendəʊkrɪˈnɒlədʒɪ/	study of the endocrine glands 内分泌学
		crinogenic /krɪnəˈdʒenɪk/	causing secretion 促分泌的
end/o	inside, internal 内	endogenous /enˈdɒdʒɪnəs/	originating from the inside 内生的
		endoscope /ˈendəskəʊp/	instrument to view the inside of the body 内镜
ex/o	out, external 外	exocrine /ˈeksəʊkraɪn/	(gland) that secretes externally 外分泌（腺）
		exogenous /ekˈsɒdʒɪnəs/	originating from the outside 外生的

Continue

Word Part	Meaning	Example Term	Meaning in English and Chinese
gluc/o	sugar 糖；glucose 葡萄糖	glucogenesis /ˌgluːkəʊˈdʒenɪsɪs/	production of glucose 葡萄糖生成
		glucolysis /gluːˈkɒlɪsɪs/	breaking down of the glucose 糖解
glyc/o	sugar 糖	glycopenia /glaɪkəʊˈpiːnɪə/	deficiency of sugar in tissue 低血糖
		hyperglycemia /ˌhaɪpəgləˈsiːmɪə/	high level of sugar in blood 高血糖症
gonad/o	gonad, sex gland 性腺	hypergonadism /haɪpəˈgɒnædɪzəm/	overactivity of the sex gland 性腺功能亢进
		gonadopathy /gɒnəˈdɒpəθɪ/	disease of the gonads 性腺病
hormon/o	hormone 激素	hormonal /hɔːˈməʊnl/	pertaining to hormone 激素的
		hormonogenesis /ˌhɔːmənəʊˈdʒenɪsɪs/	formation of hormones 激素生成
mamm/o	breast 乳房	mammoplasty /ˈmæməʊˌplæstɪ/	surgical repair of the breast 乳房成形术
		mammotomy /mæˈmɒtəmɪ/	incision into the breast 乳房切开术
medull/o	medulla 脊髓	medulloblast /mɪˈdʌləblæst/	embryonic cell of medulla 成髓细胞
		medullitis /medəˈlaɪtɪs/	inflammation of the spinal cord 脊髓炎
pancreat/o	pancreas 胰腺	pancreatic /ˌpæŋkrɪˈætɪk/	pertaining to the pancreas 胰腺的
		pancreatogram /ˌpæŋkrɪˈætəgræm/	X-ray image of the pancreas 胰造影图
parathyroid/o	parathyroid gland 甲状旁腺	parathyroidectomy /ˌpærəˌθaɪrɔɪˈdektəmɪ/	excision of a parathyroid gland 甲状旁腺切除术
		hypoparathyroidism /ˌhaɪpəˌpærəˈθaɪrɔɪdɪzm/	underactivity of the parathyroid glands 甲状旁腺功能减退
pineal/o	pineal gland 松果腺	pinealism /pɪˈnɪəlɪzəm/	abnormal activity of the pineal body 松果体功能障碍
		pinealoma /pɪnɪəˈləʊmə/	tumor of the pineal gland 松果体瘤
pituit/o	pituitary 垂体	pituitectomy /pɪˌtjuːɪˈtektəmɪ/	removal of pituitary gland 垂体切除术
		hyperpituitarism /ˌhaɪpəpɪˈtjuːɪtərɪzəm/	overactivity of the pituitary gland 垂体功能亢进
thym/o	thymus 胸腺	thymoma /θaɪˈməʊmə/	tumor of the thymus 胸腺瘤
		thymotoxic /ˌθaɪməˈtɒksɪk/	poisonous to the thymus 胸腺毒素的
thyr/o, thyroid/o	thyroid gland 甲状腺	thyrolytic /θaɪrəˈlɪtɪk/	destructive to the thyroid gland 溶甲状腺的
		thyromegaly /θaɪrəˈmegəlɪ/	enlargement of the thyroid gland 甲状腺肿大
		thyroiditis /ˌθaɪrɔɪˈdaɪtɪs/	inflammation of the thyroid gland 甲状腺炎
		hypothyroidism /ˌhaɪpəʊˈθaɪrɔɪdɪzəm/	underactivity of the thyroid gland 甲状腺功能减退

Exercises

Ⅰ. Write the definitions of the following word parts and provide an example word for each of them.

	Definition	Medical Term
1. glyc/o	sugar	glycogen
2. thyroid/o	thyroid gland	thyroiditis
3. pancreat/o	pancreas	pancreatectomy
4. calc/o	calcium	calcitonin
5. pineal/o	pineal gland	pinealoblastoma
6. adren/o	adrenal gland	adrenaline
7. end/o	inside, internal	endocrinology
8. hormon/o	hormone	hormonotherapy

Ⅱ. Explain the meaning of the following medical terms.

1. hypopituitarism   underactivity of the pituitary gland
2. thyroidectomy   removal of the thyroid gland
3. pancreatomegaly   enlargement of the pancreas
4. hypoglycemia   low levels of sugar in blood
5. hormonology   study of the hormones
6. adenomalacia   softening of the gland
7. mammectomy   removal of the breast
8. endocellular   pertaining to inside the cell

Ⅲ. Match each word part in Column A with its English term in Column B. Write the corresponding letter in the blank provided.

Column A		Column B
_D_	1. pituit/o	A. male
_E_	2. thyr/o	B. sugar
_A_	3. andr/o	C. thymus
_I_	4. hormon/o	D. pituitary gland
_J_	5. gluc/o	E. thyroid gland
_G_	6. parathyroid/o	F. breast
_C_	7. thym/o	G. parathyroid gland
_H_	8. gonad/o	H. gonad
_F_	9. mamm/o	I. hormone
_B_	10. glyc/o	J. glucose

Section B   Reading Passages

Passage one   The Endocrine System

Exercises

I. Define the following endocrine glands of the human body and translate them into Chinese.

1. hypothalamus	a region of the brain between the thalamus and the midbrain	下丘脑
2. pineal gland	a small, cone-shaped endocrine gland in the brain	松果腺
3. pituitary gland	a small, somewhat cherry-shaped double structure attached by a stalk to the base of the brain	（脑）垂体
4. thyroid gland	a two-lobed endocrine gland, located at the base of the neck that secretes two hormones that regulate the rates of metabolism, growth, and development	甲状腺
5. thymus gland	a ductless, butterfly-shaped gland lying at the base of the neck, formed mostly of lymphatic tissue and aiding in the production of T cells of the immune system	胸腺
6. adrenal gland	one of a pair of ductless glands, located above the kidneys, consisting of a cortex and a medulla	肾上腺
7. pancreas	a gland, situated near the stomach, that secretes a digestive fluid into the intestine through one or more ducts and also secretes the hormone insulin	胰腺
8. ovary	the female gonad or reproductive gland, in which the ova and the hormones that regulate female secondary sex characteristics develop	卵巢
9. testis	the male gonad or reproductive gland, either of two oval glands located in the scrotum	睾丸

II. Match each word in Column A with its definition in Column B. Write the corresponding letter in the blank provided.

	Column A	Column B
F	1. pineal	A. hormone secreted by the adrenal medulla
J	2. thyroid	B. the soft, marrow-like center of an organ
H	3. melatonin	C. outer section of an organ
I	4. endocrinology	D. two to three pairs of pea-shaped organs located on the back of the thyroid gland
A	5. adrenaline	E. hormone secreted by the pancreas
C	6. cortex	F. a small gland located deep in the brain

___E___ 7. glucagon   G. male hormone produced by the testes

___B___ 8.medulla   H. hormone produced by the pineal gland

___D___ 9. parathyroid glands   I. study of the endocrine glands

___G___ 10. testosterone   J. an endocrine gland on either side of the larynx and upper trachea

Ⅲ.Translate the following into English.

1. 皮质	cortex	2. 肾上腺	adrenal gland
3. 甲状腺	thyroid	4. 甲状旁腺	parathyroid
5. 胸腺	thymus gland	6. 固醇	sterol
7. 外分泌腺	exocrine gland	8. 内分泌腺	endocrine gland
9. 下丘脑	hypothalamus	10.去甲肾上腺素	noradrenaline
11.卵巢激素	ovarian hormone	12.睾酮	testosterone

Ⅳ.Fill in each blank with a proper word or words.

The endocrine system, along with the nervous system, functions in the regulation of body activities. The nervous system acts through (1) electrical impulses and neurotransmitters to cause muscle contraction and (2) glandular secretion. The effect is of short duration, measured in seconds, and localized. The endocrine system acts through chemical messengers called (3) hormones that influence growth, development, and metabolic activities. The action of the endocrine system is (4) measured in minutes, hours, or weeks and is more generalized than the action of the nervous system.

The endocrine glands do not have (5) ducts to carry their product to a surface. They are called ductless glands. The word endocrine is derived from the Greek terms "endo", meaning (6) within, and "krine", meaning to separate or (7) secrete. The secretory products of endocrine glands are called hormones and are secreted directly into the (8) blood and then carried throughout the body where they influence only those cells that have (9) receptor sites for that hormone.

Passage Two   Endocrine Disorders

Exercises

Ⅰ. Define the diagnostic terms about endocrine system in Column A with the descriptions in Column B. Write the corresponding letter in the blank provided.

Column A	Column B
___I___ 1. acromegaly	A. excessive potassium in the blood
___B___ 2. adrenalitis	B. inflammation of an adrenal gland
___C___ 3. adrenomegaly	C. enlargement of the adrenal glands
___E___ 4. hypercalcemia	D. state of deficient thyroid gland activity
___F___ 5. hyperglycemia	E. excessive calcium in the blood
___A___ 6. hyperkalemia	F. excessive sugar in the blood

G	7. hyperthyroidism	G. state of excessive production of the thyroid hormone
J	8. hypoglycemia	H. tumor of the parathyroid gland
D	9. hypothyroidism	I. enlargement of the extremities
H	10. parathyroidoma	J. deficient level of sugar in the blood

Ⅱ. Translate the following into Chinese.

1. hypersecretion	分泌过多	2. anabolism	合成代谢
3. catabolism	分解代谢	4. acromegaly	肢端肥大症
5. polyuria	多尿症	6. polydipsia	烦渴
7. goiter	甲状腺肿	8. tachycardia	心动过速
9. exophthalmos	眼球突出症	10. thyroidectomy	甲状腺切除术
11. dehydration	脱水	12. ketoacidosis	酮症酸中毒

Ⅲ. Translate the following into English.

Hormone levels that are too high or too low indicate a problem with the endocrine system. Hormone-related diseases occur if your body does not respond to hormones in the appropriate ways. Stress, infection, and changes in the blood fluid and electrolyte balance can also influence hormone levels, according to the USA National Institutes of Health (NIH).

The most common endocrine disease in the United States is diabetes, a condition in which the body does not properly process glucose, a simple sugar. This is due to the lack of insulin or, if the body is producing insulin, the body is not working effectively.

Ⅳ. Discuss the following topics.

1. Describe the usual signs and symptoms seen in endocrine disorders.

   The following signs and symptoms are frequently seen in patients with endocrine diseases. Weight changes, either gains or losses, are an expression of the hormonal effects on metabolic processes, so-called anabolism and catabolism, skin, hair, and nail changes can be part of an increased catabolic state. Excess production of these hormones in patients with Cushing syndrome, primary aldosteronism, and pheochromocytoma is associated with hypertension. On the other hand, hypotension is seen in patients with cortisol deficiency, hypoaldosteronism, or sympathetic dysfunction. Hormones affect energy and muscle function. Their deficiency may lead to weakness and tiredness. Since the female menstrual cycle is greatly influenced by gonadotropins, estrogen, and other hormones, menstrual irregularities are common manifestations of endocrine dysfunction.

2. What are the better ways to avoid endocrine disorders?

   The answer is open.

3. Give a brief description of the symptoms of Cushing syndrome and Addison disease.

   Symptoms of Cushing syndrome include hypertension, weakness, hyperglycemia, excess hair growth in females, and a peculiar obesity limited to the face, neck and trunk.

Weight loss, low blood pressure, and electrolyte imbalance, weakness, and increased pigmentation of the skin are symptoms of Addison disease.

Passage Three   Hypoglycemia

Exercises

Ⅰ. Read the following statements and decide whether they are true or false. Then write T for true and F for false in the brackets.

[T] 1. Since the brain depends almost exclusively on glucose metabolism to satisfy its energy requirements, brain function is disrupted by even brief periods of glucose deprivation.

[T] 2. Hypoglycemia is a condition related to disordered fuel homeostasis.

[F] 3. In fuel metabolism, the anabolic phase is characterized by falling insulin levels and rising levels of four counterregulatory hormones.

[F] 4. Hepatic gluconeogenesis derives both from carbohydrate and noncarbohydrate substrates.

[T] 5. The fall of insulin levels and the rise in the four counterregulatory hormones are needed to defend against hypoglycemia.

[F] 6. Hypoglycemia occurring solely in the fed state is most generally functional and does not pose a threat to the health of a patient.

[T] 7. Insulin overdose is probably the most frequent cause of hypoglycemia.

[F] 8. Drug-induced hypoglycemia is most likely to be seen in the sick and the aged.

Ⅱ. Here is a list of terms from the text. Analyze their meanings using the word building knowledge you have learned. Leave the space empty if the word part does not apply.

Term	Prefix	Root	Suffix	Chinese Translation
1. gluconeogenesis		gluco- neo- gen-	-sis	糖（原）异生（作用）
2. gastrectomy		gastro-	-ectomy	胃切除术
3. galactosemia		galacto-	-emia	半乳糖血症
4. gastrojejunostomy		gastro- jejuno-	-stomy	胃空肠吻合术
5. pyloroplasty		pyloro-	-plasty	幽门成形术
6. neuroglycopenia		neuro- glyco-	-penia	神经低血糖症
7. hypoglycemia	hypo-	glyco-	-emia	低血糖症

Chapter Three Urinary System

 ## Section A Medical Terminology

Learn the following combining forms, prefixes and suffixes for the urinary system and try to write in the blank space the literal meaning both in English and Chinese of the supplied terminology.

Word Part	Meaning	Example Term	Meaning in English and Chinese
cyst/o, vesic/o	sac 囊；urinary bladder 膀胱	cystography /sɪsˈtɒɡrəfɪ/	process of recording the X-ray image of the urinary bladder 膀胱造影术
		cystitis /sɪsˈtaɪtɪs/	inflammation of the urinary bladder 膀胱炎
		vesicocele /ˈvesɪkəʊsiːl/	protrusion of the bladder 膀胱膨出
		vesicotomy /ˌvesɪˈkɒtəmɪ/	incision into urinary bladder 膀胱切开术
dips/o	thirst 渴	dipsotherapy /dɪpsəʊˈθerəpɪ/	treatment through limiting the amount of fluids ingested 限饮疗法
		dipsogen /ˈdɪpsəʊdʒən/	an agent that causes thirst 致渴剂
glomerul/o	glomerulus 肾小球	glomerulonephritis /ɡlɒˌmerjʊləʊnefˈraɪtɪs/	inflammation of renal glomeruli 肾小球性肾炎
		glomerular /ɡlɒˈmerjʊlə/	pertaining to glomerulus 肾小球的
keton/o	ketone 酮	ketonuria /kiːtəʊˈnjʊərɪə/	presence of ketone in urine 酮尿
		ketonemia /kiːtəʊˈniːmɪə/	presence of ketone in blood 酮血症
meat/o	opening, canal 道，口	meatus /mɪˈeɪtəs/	external opening of a canal [解剖]道
		meatorrhaphy /mɪæˈtɒrəfɪ/	surgical suture of the meatus 尿道口缝合术
nephr/o, ren/o	kidney 肾	nephritis /neˈfraɪtɪs/	inflammation of the kidney 肾炎
		nephrectomy /neˈfrektəmɪ/	excision of the kidney 肾切除术
		renal /ˈriːnəl/	relating to the kidney 肾脏的
		renipuncture /renɪˈpʌŋktʃər/	surgical puncture of the kidney 肾穿刺术

Continue

Word Part	Meaning	Example Term	Meaning in English and Chinese
noct/i	night 夜	noctiphobia /nɒktɪˈfəubjə/	fear of night and darkness 黑夜恐怖症
		nocturnal /nɒkˈtɜːrnl/	pertaining to the night 夜的
olig/o	scanty, few 少，寡	oliguria /ɒlɪˈgjuərɪə/	scanty urination 少尿
		oligopepsia /ɒlɪgəuˈpepsɪə/	inadequate digestion 消化力不足
-pexy	surgical fixation 固定术	ovariopexy /ˌəuværɪəuˈpeksɪ/	surgical fixation of the ovary 卵巢固定术
		uteropexy /juːtərəuˈpeksɪ/	surgical fixation of the uterus 子宫固定术
-ptosis	falling or downward displacement of an organ 下垂	nephroptosis /nefrɒpˈtəusɪs/	falling of the kidney 肾下垂
		cystoptosis /ˌsɪstɒpˈtəusɪs/	downward displacement of the urinary bladder 膀胱下垂
pyel/o	renal pelvis 肾盂	pyelogram /ˈpaɪələugræm/	the X-ray image of renal pelvis 肾盂造影照片
		pyelometry /paɪˈlɒmɪtrɪ/	the process of measuring renal pelvis 骨盆测量法
retro-	behind, backward 后，向后	retrocervical /ˌretrəuˈsɜːvɪkl/	behind the cervix uteri 子宫颈后的
		retrosternal /ˌretrəuˈstɜːnl/	behind the sternum 胸骨后的
-rrhaphy	surgical suture 缝合术	urethrorrhaphy /juəreθˈrɒrəfɪ/	surgical suture of the urethra 尿道缝合术
		cystorrhaphy /sɪsˈtɔːrəfɪ/	surgical suture of the bladder 膀胱缝合术
-sclerosis	hardening 硬化	atherosclerosis /ˌæθərəuˌskləˈrɒsɪs/	hardening of the inside of blood vessels 动脉粥样硬化
		angiosclerosis /ˌændʒɪəuskləˈrɒsɪs/	hardening of the blood vessels 血管硬化
trans-	through 穿过，经过	transurethral /ˌtrænsjuˈrɪθrəl/	through the urethra 经尿道的
		transabdominal /ˌtrænsæbˈdɒmɪnəl/	through the abdomen 经腹的
trigon/o	trigone, triangle 三角，三角区	trigonitis /traɪgəˈnaɪtɪs/	inflammation of the vesical trigone 膀胱三角炎
		trigonum /traɪˈgəunəm/	a three-cornered object or area 三角区
ureter/o	ureter 输尿管	ureterostenosis /juˌriːtərɒsteˈnəusɪs/	narrowing of a ureter 输尿管狭窄
		ureterolithotomy /juˌriːtərəulɪˈθɒtəmɪ/	incision of a ureter to remove calculus 输尿管石切除术

Continue

Word Part	Meaning	Example Term	Meaning in English and Chinese
urethr/o	urethra 尿道	urethroscope /jʊˈriːθrə،skəʊp/	an instrument to view into the urethra 尿道镜
		urethrodynia /jʊ،riːθrəˈdɪnɪə/	pain in the urethra 尿道痛
-uria	urine condition 尿况	pyuria /paɪˈjʊərɪə/	presence of pus in urine 脓尿
		dysuria /dɪsˈjʊərɪə/	painful or difficult urination 排尿困难

Exercises

Ⅰ. Write the definitions of the following combining forms in English and Chinese.

Combining Form	English Meaning	Chinese Meaning
1. sclerosis	hardening	硬化
2. glomerul/o	glomerulus	肾小球
3. ket/o	ketones	酮
4. retr/o	behind	后，向后
5. nephr/o	kidney	肾
6. noct/i	night	夜
7. pyel/o	renal pelvis	肾盂
8. ren/o	kidney	肾

Ⅱ. Write the combining form(s) for each of the following words.

English Meaning	Combining Form	Chinese Meaning
1. trigone	trigon/o	三角，三角区
2. urine	urin/o, ur/o	尿
3. ureter	ureter/o	输尿管
4. scanty	olig/o	少，寡
5. opening	meat/o	道，口
6. surgical fixation	-pexy	固定术
7. surgical suture	-rrhaphy	缝合术
8. thirst	dips/o	渴
9. urethra	urethr/o	尿道
10. kidney	ren/o, nephr/o	肾

Ⅲ. Match the abnormal disorders in Column A with the correct definitions in Column B. Write the corresponding letter in the blank provided.

	Column A	Column B
F	1. cystoptosis	A. causing thirst
G	2. noctiphobia	B. inadequate digestion

A	3. dipsogenic	C. hardening of the gland
E	4. nephropathy	D. surgical suture of the urinary bladder
B	5. oligopepsia	E. disease of the kidney
C	6. adenosclerosis	F. downward displacement of the urinary bladder
D	7. cystorrhaphy	G. fear of the night and darkness
J	8. urethrodynia	H. difficult urination
H	9. dysuria	I. protrusion of the urinary bladder
I	10. vesicocele	J. pain in the urethra

➜ Section B   Reading Passages

Passage one   Common Knowledge of the Urinary System

Exercises

Ⅰ. Fill in the blanks with the correct terms.

A. urethra	B. acidosis	C. glomerulus
D. bilirubinuria	E. pyuria	F. angiotensin
G. glycosuria	H. arteriole	I. Bowman capsule

1. Excessive blood acidity caused by an overabundance of acid in the blood (B)
2. Any of several vasoconstrictor substances that cause narrowing of blood vessels (F)
3. The condition of urine containing white blood cells or pus (E)
4. A condition characterized by an excess of sugar in the urine, typically associated with diabetes or kidney disease (G)
5. An abnormality where conjugated bilirubin is detected in the urine (D)
6. A small intertwined group of capillaries (C)
7. A tube that connects the urinary bladder to the urinary meatus for the removal of fluids from the body (A)
8. A double-walled, cup-shaped structure around the glomerulus of each nephron (I)
9. A small blood vessel that forms a connection between small arteries and capillaries (H)

Ⅱ. Match the word or expression in Column A with its description in Column B. Write the corresponding letter in the blank provided.

Column A	Column B
C 1. ureter	A. a hormone secreted by the kidney that stimulates formation of red blood cells
I 2. trigone	B. notch on the surface of the kidney where blood vessels and nerve enter
J 3. renal cortex	C. tube that carries urine from the kidney to the bladder

H	4. renal medulla	D. nitrogenous waste
D	5. urea	E. cup-like collecting region of the renal pelvis
A	6. erythropoietin	F. a small molecule that carries an electric charge in solution
G	7. glomerulus	G. little ball-shaped cluster of capillaries located at the top of each nephron
F	8. electrolyte	H. substance made by the kidney that causes blood pressure to rise
B	9. hilum	I. triangular area in the bladder
E	10. calyx	J. outer section of the kidney

Ⅲ.Translate the following anatomical terms into English.

1. 输尿管	ureter	2. 腹腔	abdominal (peritoneal) cavity
3. 膀胱	urinary bladder	4. 皮质	cortex
5. 尿道	urethral meatus	6. 尿素	urea
7. 肾门	hilum of kidney	8. 髓质	medulla
9. 肾小管	renal tubule	10.盆腔	pelvic cavity

Ⅳ.Answer the following questions.

1. What is the urinary system made up of?

The urinary system is made up of two kidneys, two ureters, urinary bladder and urethra. The two kidneys are bean-shaped organs situated behind the abdominal cavity, retroperitoneal, on either side of the vertebral column in the lumbar region of the spine; the two ureters are muscular tubes lined with mucous membrane; the urinary bladder is a hollow, muscular, distensible sac in the pelvic cavity; the urethra is membranous tube through which urine is discharged from the urinary bladder.

2. How is urine formed?

As blood passes through the glomeruli, the process of forming urine begins. There are three steps to this process: filtration, reabsorption, and secretion. The walls of the glomeruli are thin enough to permit water, salts, sugar, and nitrogenous wastes such as urea, creatinine, and uric acid to filter out of the blood. Each glomerulus is surrounded by a cup-like structure that collects the substances filtering out of the blood. Each Bowman's capsule is connected to a long, twisted tube called the renal tubule. As the water, salts, sugar, and wastes pass along the tubule, the materials that the body needs i.e. most water, salts, and sugar, are able to reenter the bloodstream through tiny capillaries that lie close to each renal tubule. Thus, by the time the filtrated material reaches the end of the renal tubule, the materials that the body must keep have been reabsorbed into the bloodstream. Only the wastes, along with some water, some salts i.e. electrolytes, and some acids, pass from the renal tubule into the central collecting area of the kidney. Here, thousands of renal tubules deposit urine into the central renal pelvis, a space that fills most of the medulla of the kidney.

3. What are often tested in urinalysis?

They are color, pH, protein, glucose, specific gravity, ketone bodies, pus and bilirubin.

4. What should we do to keep our urinary system healthy?

   The answer is open.

Passage Two   Disorders of the Urinary System and Some Means for Finding Them out

Exercises

Ⅰ. Write a medical word for each of the following definitions.

1. multicapsular	polycystic
2. an examination of the inside of the bladder	cystoscope
3. a collection of pus that has built up within the tissue	abscess
4. outside the body	extracorporeal
5. crushing of stones	lithotripsy
6. removing waste and excess water from the blood	dialysis
7. a sexually transmitted infection	gonorrhea
8. a surgical method for removal of calculi	lithotomy
9. class of bacteria including Chlamydiaceae	chlamydia
10. of the lining of the abdominal cavity	peritoneal

Ⅱ. Translate the following disorders of the urinary system into English.

1. 膀胱炎	cystitis
2. 肾小球肾炎	glomerulonephritis
3. 急性肾衰竭	acute renal failure
4. 结石病	uninary lithiasis
5. 血尿症	hematuria
6. 尿毒症	uremia
7. 肾绞痛	renal colic
8. 肾盂积水	hydronephrosis
9. 尿滞留	urinary stasis
10. 蛋白尿	proteinuria

Ⅲ. Fill in the following blanks with one proper word.

The urinary system, also known as the renal system, produces, stores and eliminates urine, the fluid waste excreted by the kidneys. The kidneys make urine by (1) filtering wastes and extra water from blood. Urine travels from the kidneys through ureters and (2) fills the bladder. When the bladder is full, a person (3) urinates through the urethra to eliminate the waste.

Kidney stones are clumps of calcium oxalate that can be found anywhere in the urinary tract. Kidney stones form when chemicals in the urine become (4) concentrated enough to form a solid mass. They can cause (5) pain in the back and sides, as well as blood in the urine. Kidney failure, also called (6) renal failure and chronic kidney disease, can be a temporary (often acute) condition or can become a chronic condition resulting in the (7) <u>inability</u> of the kidneys to filter waste from the blood. Other conditions, such as diabetes and hypertension, can cause (8) <u>chronic</u> kidney disease. Acute cases may be caused by trauma or other damage, and may improve over time with (9) <u>treatment</u>. However, renal disease may lead to chronic kidney failure, which may require dialysis treatments or even a (10) <u>kidney</u> transplant.

Ⅳ.Discuss the following topics.

1. What are the causes of cystitis?

   Cystitis is an infection of the urinary bladder. Organisms generally enter through the urethra and ascend toward the bladder. The infecting organisms are usually colon bacteria carried in feces. Cystitis is thus more common in females than in males because the female urethra is shorter than the male urethra and its opening is closer to the anus. Poor toilet habits and urinary stasis are contributing factors.

2. What are the causes of acute renal failure?

   An injury, shock, exposure to toxins, infections, and other renal disorders may cause damage to the nephrons resulting in acute renal failure.

3. Describe the procedure of hemodialysis.

   In hemodialysis, blood is cleansed by passage over a membrane surrounded by fluid (dialysate) that draws out unwanted substances. In peritoneal dialysis, fluid is introduced into the peritoneal cavity. This fluid is periodically withdrawn along with waste products and replaced. This may be done at intervals throughout the day in continuous ambulatory peritoneal dialysis or at night in continuous cyclic peritoneal dialysis.

Passage Three Uremia

Exercises

Ⅰ. Read the following statements and decide whether they are true or false. Then write T for true and F for false in the brackets.

[F] 1. Uremia contains various syndromes which is the end stage of one kidney disease.

[T] 2. In the end of uremia, most systems in the body will be affected.

[F] 3. Uremia can cause heart failure, psychosis and urinary tract obstruction.

[F] 4. Patients should eat less halibut, mussels, scallops and oysters because there is poor cadmium in them.

[T] 5. Syndromes in gastrointestinal tracts are the initial manifestations of the patients with uremia.

[T] 6. Although uremia affects all systems, disorders of water and electrolyte and metabolic imbalance of protein, carbohydrate, fat and vitamin are most common.

[F] 7. Dialysis and kidney transplant addresses uremia permanently.

[F] 8. Immunotherapy is the best in treating renal disease today.

[F] 9. The patients should avoid food rich in protein and calcium to keep away from nitremia.

[T] 10. Without proper treatment, the prognosis of uremia is poor.

II. Here is a list of terms from the text. Analyze their meanings using the word building knowledge you have learned. Leave the space empty if the word part does not apply.

Term	Prefix	Root	Suffix	Chinese Translation
1. glomerulonephritis		glomerul/o nephr/i	-itis	肾小球肾炎
2. pyelonephritis		pyel/o nephr/i	-itis	肾盂肾炎
3. arteriosclerosis		arteri/o scler-	-osis	动脉硬化
4. pericarditis	peri-	cardi	-itis	心包炎
5. bronchitis		bronchi	-itis	支气管炎

Chapter Four Reproductive System

 Section A Medical Terminology

Learn the following combining forms, prefixes and suffixes for the reproductive system and try to write in the blank space the literal meaning both in English and Chinese of the provided terminology.

Word Part	Meaning	Example Term	Meaning in English and Chinese
cervic/o	uterine cervix 子宫颈；neck 颈	cervicovesical /ˌsɜːvɪkəu'vesɪkəl/	pertaining to the uterine cervix and the bladder 子宫颈膀胱的
		cervicitis /sɜːvɪ'saɪtɪs/	inflammation of the uterine cervix 子宫颈炎
chori/o	chorionic membrane 绒（毛）膜	choriogenesis /ˌkəurɪə'dʒenəsɪs/	the development of the chorion 绒毛膜发生
		chorioma /kəurɪ'əumə/	tumor of chorion 绒毛膜瘤
colp/o	vagina 阴道	colpatresia /ˌkɒlpə'triːzɪə/	occlusion of the vagina 阴道闭锁
		colpectasia /ˌkɒlpek'teɪzɪə/	dilation of the vagina 阴道扩张
-cyesis	pregnancy 妊娠（期）	pseudocyesis /sjuːdəusaɪ'iːsɪs/	false pregnancy 假孕
		acyesis /æsɪ'iːsɪs/	absence of pregnancy 不孕
epididym/o	epididymis 附睾	epididymectomy /ˌepɪdɪdɪ'mektəmɪ/	excision of epididymis 附睾切除术
		epididymotomy /ˌepɪdɪdɪ'mɒtəmɪ/	incision of the epididymis 附睾切开术
episi/o	vulva 外阴，女阴	episiotomy /ˌepɪsɪ'ɒtəmɪ/	incision of the vulva 外阴切开术
		episiorrhaphy /ˌepɪsɪ'ɒrəfɪ/	surgical suture of the vulva 外阴缝合术
galact/o	milk 乳；milk gland 乳腺	galactorrhea /gəˌlæktəu'riːə/	overflow of breast milk 乳溢
		galactoma /gælæk'təumə/	swelling of the milk gland 乳腺囊肿
hyster/o, metr/o	uterus, womb 子宫	hysterectomy /ˌhɪstə'rektəmɪ/	removal of the uterus 子宫切除
		hysterocele /'hɪstərəusiːl/	hernia of the uterus 子宫疝
		metroptosis /ˌmetrəu'ptəusɪs/	downward displacement of the uterus 子宫脱垂
		metroplasty /ˌmetrəu'plæstɪ/	surgical repair of the uterus 子宫成形术

Continue

Word Part	Meaning	Example Term	Meaning in English and Chinese
lact/o	milk 乳	lactogenesis /ˌlæktə'dʒenəsɪs/	production of milk 乳汁生成
		lactic /'læktɪk/	relating to milk 乳汁的
men/o	menstruation, menses 月经	menorrhagia /ˌmenə'reɪdʒɪə/	excessive menses 月经过多
		dysmenorrhea /ˌdɪsmenə'rɪə/	painful menstruation 痛经
myom/o	muscle tumor 肌瘤	myomotomy /maɪə'mɔːtəmɪ/	incision of a muscle tumor 肌瘤切开术
		myomectomy /maɪə'mektəmɪ/	surgical removal of muscle tumor 肌瘤切除术
orchi/o, orchid/o, test/o	testicle 睾丸	orchidopexy /ˌɔːkɪdəu'peksɪ/	surgical fixation of an undescended testis 睾丸固定术
		orchiectomy /ɔːkɪ'ektəmɪ/	excision of a testis 睾丸切除术
		testalgia /tes'tældʒɪə/	pain of the testis 睾丸痛
		testitis /tes'taɪtɪs/	inflammation of the testis 睾丸炎
oophor/o, ovari/o	ovary 卵巢	oophorectomy /ˌəufə'rektəmɪ/	excision of the ovary 卵巢切除术
		oophoropexy / ˌəufərəu'peksɪ/	surgical fixation of the ovary 卵巢固定术
		ovariopathy /əuˌvaːrɪ'ɒpəsɪ/	disease of the ovary 卵巢病
		ovariocentesis /əuˌvaːrɪə'sentiːsɪs /	surgical puncture into an ovary 卵巢穿刺术
o/o, ov/i	egg 卵	oogenesis /əuə'dʒenɪsɪs/	development of an egg 卵子发生
		oocyte/ 'əuəsaɪt/	an egg cell 卵细胞
		oviform /'əuvɪfɔːm/	in the form of an egg 卵形的
		ovicide /'əuvɪsaɪd/	an agent that kills eggs 杀卵剂
prostat/o	prostate gland 前列腺	prostatolith /'prɒsteɪtəˌlɪθ/	stone in the prostate gland 前列腺结石
		prostatotomy /ˌprɒstə'tɒtəmɪ/	incision of the prostate 前列腺切开术
salping/o	uterine tube, oviduct 输卵管	salpingopexy /ˌsælpɪŋəu'peksɪ/	fixation of a uterine tube 输卵管固定术
		salpingocyesis /ˌsælpɪŋəusaɪ'ɪsɪs/	pregnancy within a uterine tube 输卵管妊娠
sperm/o, spermat/o	sperm 精子, 精液	oligospermia /ɒlɪgəu'spəmɪə/	scanty sperm 精子减少
		spermatolysis /ˌspɜːmə'tɒlɪsɪs/	breaking down of sperm 精子溶解
terat/o	monster 怪物; malformed 畸形	teratoma /ˌterə'təumə/	a tumor consisting of foreign tissues 畸胎瘤
		teratospermia /te'raːtəuspəmɪə/	malformed sperm in semen 畸形精子

Continue

Word Part	Meaning	Example Term	Meaning in English and Chinese
-tocia	labor, birth 分娩	dystocia /dɪsˈtəʊʃɪə/	difficult labor 难产
		eutocia /juˈtəʊʃɪə/	normal childbirth 正常分娩
vulv/o	vulva 女阴；external genitalia 外阴	vulvocleisis /vʌlvəˈklaɪsɪs/	surgical closure of the vulva 外阴闭合术
		vulvitis /vʌlˈvaɪtɪs/	inflammation of the vulva 外阴炎

Exercises

Ⅰ. Write the definitions of the following combining forms in English and Chinese and then provide an example term containing the combining form.

Combining Form	English Meaning	Chinese Meaning	Example Term
1. vulv/o	vulva, external genetalia	外阴，女阴	vulvopathy
2. salping/o	oviduct	输卵管	salpingocele
3. galact/o	milk, milk gland	乳，乳腺	galactoma
4. oophor/o	ovary	卵巢	oophoroma
5. o/o	egg	卵	ooblast
6. ov/o	egg	卵	ovocyte
7. myom/o	muscle tumor	肌瘤	myomotomy
8. metr/o	uterus	子宫	metropexy

Ⅱ. Write a combining form for each of the following terms and then provide an example term containing the combining form.

Word	Combining Form	Example Term
1. menstruation	men/o 月经	menopause 绝经
2. milk	lact/o 乳	lactogenic 生乳的
3. uterus	hyster/o 子宫	hysterometry 子宫测量法
4. labor, birth	-tocia 分娩	dystocia 难产
5. vagina	colp/o 阴道	colpedema 阴道水肿
6. cervix	cervic/o 子宫颈	cervicitis 子宫颈炎
7. epididymis	epididym/o 附睾	epididymotomy 附睾切开术
8. testis	test/o 睾丸	testosterone 睾丸素，睾酮

Ⅲ. Match the terms in Column A with their definitions in Column B. Write the corresponding letter in the blank provided.

Column A	Column B
__E__ 1. spermatogenesis	A. inflammation of the testes
__D__ 2. prostatitis	B. inflammation of the epididymis
__B__ 3. epididymitis	C. excision of the prostate gland

F	4. orchiopexy	D.	inflammation of the prostate gland
C	5. prostatectomy	E.	the formation of sperm cells
A	6. orchitis	F.	fixation of an undescended testicle
G	7. oligospermia	G.	scanty sperm
J	8. hysteropathy	H.	without sperm
I	9. testicular	I.	pertaining to a testicle
H	10. aspermia	J.	disease of the womb

→ Section B   Reading Passages

Passage One   The Reproductive System

Exercises

Ⅰ. Write a word for each of the following definitions.

1. the regular discharge of blood and mucosal tissue from the uterus   menstruation

2. two very fine tubes leading from the ovaries into the uterus   fallopian tube

3. the first menstrual cycle   menarche

4. the time when menstrual cycle ends   menopause

5. a temporary endocrine structure in female ovaries   corpus luteum

6. an organic fluid that may contain spermatozoa   semen

7. the external genital organs of a woman   vulva

8. the release of egg from the ovaries   ovulation

Ⅱ. Translate the following terms into English.

1. 生殖器官   reproductive organ

2. 附属器官   accessory organ

3. 外生殖器   external genitalia

4. 前列腺   prostate gland

5. 尿道球腺（考珀腺）   bulbourethral gland (Cowper's gland)

6. 乳腺   mammary gland

7. 输精管   vas deferens

8. 输卵管   fallopian tube

Ⅲ. Write the plural forms of the following singular terms.

1. ovum   ova

2. endometrium   endometria

3. myometrium   myometria

4. perimetrium   perimetria

5. fundus   fundi

6. uterus   uteri/uteruses
7. focus   foci/focuses
8. anus   anus(es)
9. testis   testes
10. meiosis   meioses
11. alkalosis   alkaloses
12. ecchymosis   ecchymoses
13. spermatozoon   spermatozoa
14. protozoon   protozoa
15. anthozoon   anthozoa
16. neutron   neutrons
17. cervix   cervices/cervixes
18. matrix   matrices/matrixes
19. apex   apices/apexes
20. codex   codices
21. chlamydia   chlamydiae
22. formula   formulae/formulas
23. axilla   axillae/axillas
24. urethra   urethrae/urethras

IV.Answer the following questions.
1. What is the male reproductive system responsible for? And what are its reproductive organs?

The male reproductive or genital system is responsible for producing, transporting, and maintaining viable sperm (the male sex cell), and also produces the male sex hormone, testosterone, which regulates the development of a beard, pubic hair, a deep voice and other bodily characteristics of the adult male.

The male reproductive system consists of the testes, the ducts that transport sperm, a number of accessory glands, and the external genitalia.

2. What is the female reproductive system responsible for? And what are its reproductive organs?

The female reproductive is responsible for producing and transporting ova (the female sex cells); eliminating ova from the body, if they are not fertilized by sperm; nourishing and providing a place for growth of an embryo, if an ovum is fertilized by sperm; and nourishing a newborn child. The female reproductive system also produces the female sex hormones, estrogen and progesterone, which regulate the development of breasts and other bodily characteristics of the mature female.

The primary organs of the female reproductive system are the ovaries, fallopian tubes, uterus, vagina, and external genitalia. In addition, the mammary glands (breasts) serve as accessory organs.

3. What secretes estrogen and progesterone? And what are the functions of estrogen and progesterone?

The ovaries secrete estrogen and progesterone.

During puberty, estrogen stimulates development of secondary sex characteristics, such as increased deposition of fat in the breasts, thighs, and buttocks and the growth of pubic and axillary hair; estrogen also regulates maturation of the uterus, uterine tubes, vagina, ovaries, and breasts. In the sexually mature female, estrogen induces the process of ovulation. Progesterone secreted by the corpus luteum regulates preparation of the uterus for implantation of a fertilized ovum. During pregnancy, progesterone inhibits ovulation and causes the breasts to enlarge and secrete milk.

4. When do you think the health education about the reproductive system should start and who should educate the adolescents about the knowledge of the reproductive system?
   The answer is open.

Passage Two   Disorders of the Reproductive System

Exercises

Ⅰ. Translate the following disorders related to the reproductive system into Chinese.

1. cryptorchism   隐睾
2. testicular cancer   睾丸癌
3. hydrocele   鞘膜积液
4. gonorrhea   淋病
5. oligospermia   精子过少
6. endometriosis   子宫内膜异位
7. papilloma   乳头状瘤
8. hyperplasia   增生
9. sterility   不育
10. candidiasis   念珠菌病

Ⅱ. Describe in English the common disorders of the male and female reproductive systems.

The common disorders of the male reproductive system refer to the disorders occurring in the testes, prostate gland as well as penis. Carcinoma of the testes and carcinoma of the prostate are often life-threatening. Luckily, the hyperplasia of the prostate, epispadias, hypospadias and phimosis are curable by surgical treatment.

The common disorders of the female reproductive system include infection, endometriosis, menstrual disorders and cancers in the female reproductive tract, such as cervical carcinoma, cancer of the endometrium, cancer of the ovary and breast cancer.

Ⅲ. Fill in the blanks with one proper word.

The reproductive system is a collection of internal and external organs — in both males and females — that work together for the purpose of procreating. Due to its vital role in the survival of the species, many scientists argue that the (1) reproductive system is among the most important systems in the entire body.

The male reproductive system consists of two major parts: the testes, where (2) sperms are produced, and the penis. The penis and urethra belong to both the urinary and reproductive systems in males. The (3) testes are carried in an external pouch known as the scrotum, where they normally remain slightly cooler than body temperature to facilitate sperm production.

The external structures of the female reproductive system include the clitoris, labia (4) minora, labia (5) majora and Bartholin glands. The major (6) internal organs of the female reproductive system include the vagina and uterus — which act as the receptacle for semen — and the ovaries, which produce the female's (7) ova. The vagina is attached to the uterus through the (8) cervix, while the fallopian tubes connect the (9) uterus to the ovaries. In response to hormonal changes, one ovum, or egg — or more in the case of multiple births — is released and sent down the fallopian tube during ovulation. If not (10) fertilized, this egg is eliminated as a result of menstruation.

Ⅳ. Translate the following sentences into English.

1. 生殖系统疾病泛指影响人体生殖系统的各种疾病。

   Reproductive system disease broadly refers to any of the diseases and disorders that affect the human reproductive system.

2. 睾丸肿瘤的治疗通常包括手术治疗、放疗和化疗。

   Tumors of the testes are commonly treated with surgery, radiotherapy, and chemotherapy.

3. 前列腺癌常发生于 50 岁以上的男性中。

   Carcinoma of the prostate commonly occurs in men who are over 50 years of age.

4. 月经异常包括经量过少、经量过多和无经。

   Menstrual abnormalities include flow that is too scanty or too heavy and absence of monthly periods.

5. 对美国妇女来说，与癌症相关的死亡中，乳腺癌仅次于肺癌。

   Carcinoma of the breast is second only to lung cancer in causing cancer-related deaths among U.S. women.

Passage Three Some Basic Knowledge Related to the Reproductive System

Exercises

Ⅰ. Translate the following phrases into English.

1. 传染病   communicable disease
2. 性行为   sexual activity
3. 首发症状   initial symptom
4. 月经初潮   the onset of menstruation
5. 卵泡雌激素   follicle-stimulating hormone

6. 性交   <u>sexual intercourse</u>

7. 黄体生成素   <u>luteinizing hormone</u>

8. 阴道萎缩   <u>vaginal atrophy</u>

II. Match the abnormal conditions in Column A with their definitions in Column B. Write the corresponding letter in the blank provided.

Column A	**Column B**
_D_ 1. a disease that is contracted and transmitted by sexual contact	A. Herpes genitalis
_F_ 2. an infection of the urethra	B. Chancre
_A_ 3. a genital infection caused by the herpes simplex virus	C. Trichomoniasis
_E_ 4. a rare condition caused by transmission of herpes simplex virus from mother to newborn	D. Venereal disease
_B_ 5. a painless ulceration formed during the primary stage of syphilis	E. Neonatal herpes
_C_ 6. an infectious disease caused by the parasite trichomonal vaginitis	F. Urethritis

Chapter Five Nervous System

→ Section A Medical Terminology

Learn the following combining forms, prefixes and suffixes for the nervous system and try to write in the blank space the literal meaning both in English and Chinese of the provided terminology.

Word Part	Meaning	Example Term	Meaning in English and Chinese
cerebell/o	cerebellum 小脑	cerebellitis /ˌserəbə'laɪtɪs/	inflammation of the cerebellum 小脑炎
		cerebellospinal /ˌserəˌbelə'spaɪnl/	pertaining to the cerebellum and spinal cord 小脑脊髓的
cerebr/o	cerebrum 大脑	cerebrosclerosis /ˌserɪbrəʊsklɪə'rəʊsɪs/	hardening of the cerebrum 大脑硬化
		cerebropathy /ˌserə'brɒpəɪ/	disease of the cerebrum 大脑病
cortic/o	cortex 皮质	cortical /'kɔːtɪkl/	pertaining to the cortex 皮质的，皮层的
		corticocerebral /ˌkɔːtɪkəʊsə'rɪbrəl/	pertaining to cerebral cortex 大脑皮层的
dendr/o	dendrite 树突；	dendritic /ˌden'drɪtɪk/	pertaining to dendrite 树突的
		dendroid /'dendrɒɪd/	branching like a tree 树状的
-esthesia	feeling, sensation 感觉	hyperesthesia /ˌhaɪpəres'θiːʒɪə/	increased sensitivity 感觉过敏
		paresthesia /ˌpærəs'θiːʒɪə/	abnormal feeling 感觉异常
gli/o	glia 神经胶质	glioma /glaɪ'əʊmə/	atumor of glia 神经胶质瘤
		gliophagia /glaɪɒ'feɪdʒɪə/	eating function of glia 神经胶质细胞吞噬作用
gangli/o	ganglion 神经节	ganglioform /'gæŋglɪəˌfɔːm/	having the form of a ganglion 神经节状的
		gangliocyte /'gæŋglɪəʊˌsaɪt/	ganglion cell 神经节细胞
medull/o	medulla 髓	medulloblast /mɪ'dʌləblæst/	an immature medullary cell 成神经管细胞
		medullocell /mɪ'dʌləsel/	resembling medulla 类髓质
mening/o	meninges 脑膜；	meningocyte /'menɪngəʊˌsaɪt/	a cell of the meninges 脑膜细胞
		meningorrhagia /ˌmenɪngəʊ'rædʒɪə/	bleeding in the meninges 脑膜出血

Continue

Word Part	Meaning	Example Term	Meaning in English and Chinese
-paralysis	loss of motor function 瘫痪	hemiparalysis /hemɪpɜːˈrælɪsɪs/	paralysis of one side of the body 偏瘫
		pseudoparalysis /ˈsjuːdəupɜːˈrælɪsɪs/	false paralysis 假性瘫痪
pont/o	pons 脑桥	pontobulbia /pɒntəˈbʌlbɪə/	presence of cavities in the pons 脑桥空洞症
		pontile /ˈpɒntaɪl/	pertaining to the pons 脑桥的
-plegia	paralysis 麻痹，瘫痪	quadriplegia /ˌkwɒdrɪˈpliːdʒɪə/	paralysis of all four limbs 四肢麻痹
		paraplegia /ˌpærəˈpliːdʒɪə/	paralysis of the lower part of the body 下身麻痹
sympath/o	sympathetic nervous system 交感神经	sympatholysis /ˌsɪmpəθəuˈlɪsɪs/	excision of the sympathetic nerve 交感神经切除
		sympathoblast /sɪmˈpæθɒblæst/	embryonic cell that develops into a sympathetic nerve cell 成交感神经细胞
synapt/o	synapse 突触；神经键	synaptology /sɪnæpˈtɒlədʒɪ/	the study of synapse 突触学
		synaptolemma /saɪnæptəuˈlemə/	membrane of synapse 突触膜
thalam/o	thalamus 丘脑	thalamectomy /ˌθæləˈmektəmɪ/	removal of the thalamus 丘脑切除术
		thalamocortical /ˌθæləməˈkɔːtɪkəl/	pertaining to the thalamus and cerebral cortex 丘脑皮层的

Exercises

I. Fill in the following blanks with the terms in the box. Change the form if necessary.

cerebrosclerosis	hyperesthesia
cerebellitis	anesthesia
pseudoparalysis	meningorrhagia
paresthesia	glioma

1. Acute <u>cerebellitis</u> is a rare inflammatory process characterized by a sudden onset of cerebellar dysfunction usually affecting children. It is related as a consequence of a primary or secondary infection, or much less commonly as a result of post-vaccinal reaction.

2. The morbid hardening of the substance of the cerebrum is called <u>cerebrosclerosis</u>.

3. <u>Meningorrhagia</u> refers to the hemorrhage into or beneath the cerebral or spinal meninges.

4. A condition in which a person appears to be unable to move the arms or legs but has no "true" paralysis is called <u>pseudoparalysis</u>.

5. <u>Anesthesia</u> allows doctors to operate on patients without causing any pain.

6. <u>Paresthesia</u> is defined as an abnormal sensation of the body, such as numbness, tingling, or burning. These sensations may be felt in the fingers, hands, toes, or feet.

7. <u>Glioma</u> is a common type of primary brain tumor, accounting for about 33% of these tumors. It originates in the glial cells in the brain.

8. <u>Hyperesthesia</u> is a condition that involves an abnormal increase in sensitivity to stimuli of the sense.

Ⅱ. Match each word part in Column A with its English term in Column B. Write the corresponding letter in the blank provided.

Column A	Column B
_C_ 1. cortic/o	A. thalamus
_D_ 2. dendr/o	B. paralysis
_A_ 3. thalam/o	C. cortex
_B_ 4. -plegia	D. dendrite
_H_ 5. pont/o	E. glia
_G_ 6. mening/o	F. ganglion
_F_ 7. gangli/o	G. membrane
_E_ 8. gli/o	H. pons

Ⅲ.Write a word for each of the following definitions, using the slashes provided to separate the word elements.

1. hardening of the cerebrum   cerebr / oscler / osis
2. bleeding in the brain membranes   mening / orrhagia
3. the role of glia cells in engulfing   gli / ophagia
4. paralysis of the lower part of the body   para / plegia
5. study of the science of synapse   synapt / ology
6. surgical creation of incisions in the hypothalamus   hypo / thalam / otomy

Section B   Reading Passages

Passage One   The Nervous System

Exercises

Ⅰ. Here is a picture of the parts of a neuron and the pathway of a nervous impulse (Figure 5-1). First label it with the words in the box and then explain how impulses travel along the parts of a nerve cell.

axon	cell nucleus	synapse	dendrites
cell body	myelin sheath	terminal end fibers	

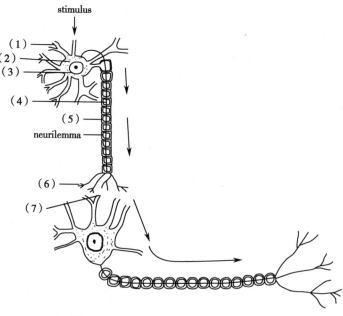

Figure 5-1   The parts of a nerve cell
(1) dendrites   (2) cell body   (3) cell nucleus   (4) axon
(5) myelin sheath   (6) terminal end fibers   (7) synapse

II. Spell out the terms according to the definitions bellow. The first letter is given to you.

1. three protective membranes that surround the brain and spinal cord   meninges
2. cells in the nervous system that do not carry impulses but are supportive and connective in function   neuroglia
3. chemical messenger, released at the end of a nerve cell, that stimulates or inhibits another cell   neurotransmitter
4. depression in the surface of the cerebral cortex; fissure   sulcus
5. nerves that carry impulses away from the brain and spinal cord to the muscles, glands, and organs; motor nerves   efferent nerves
6. tissue that surrounds the axon of some nerve fibers   myelin sheath

III. Translate the following terms into English.

1. 中枢神经系统   central nervous system   2. 周围神经系统   peripheral nervous system
3. 脑神经   cranial nerves   4. 迷走神经   vagus nerve
5. 脊神经   spinal nerves   6. 周围神经   peripheral nerves
7. 交感神经   sympathetic nerves   8. 副交感神经   parasympathetic nerves
9. 神经鞘   neurilemma   10. 神经胶质   neuroglia
11. 传出神经   efferent nerves   12. 下丘脑   hypothalamus
13. 丘脑   thalamus   14. 神经胶质细胞   neuroglial cells

Ⅳ.Answer the following questions.

1. What is the nervous system generally composed of?

   The nervous system can be classified into two major divisions: the central nervous system and the peripheral nervous system.

2. What are the major differences between the central nervous system and the peripheral nervous system?

   The central nervous system consists of the brain and spinal cord. The peripheral nervous system consists of 12 pairs of cranial nerves and 31 pairs of spinal nerves. The cranial nerves carry impulses between the brain and the head and neck. The spinal nerves carry messages between the spinal cord and the chest, abdomen, and extremities. The peripheral nervous system consists of a large group of nerves that function involuntarily or automatically without conscious control. These peripheral nerves are those of the autonomic nervous system.

3. What is gray matter and white matter?

   The gray matter refers to the collections of cell bodies and dendrites. The white matter refers to the myelin sheath.

4. What are the three layers of the meninges?

   The outermost membrane of the meninges is called the dura mater. The second layer around the brain and spinal cord is called the arachnoid membrane. The third layer of the meninges, closest to the brain and spinal cord, is called the pia mater.

Passage Two   Epilepsy

Exercises

Ⅰ. Translate the following common causes of seizures into Chinese.

1. atrophic lesions of the cerebral hemispheres　　脑半球萎缩性病变
2. problems of hypoxia in the perinatal and early antenatal period　　围产期或产前早期出现的缺氧问题
3. atrophic lesions　　萎缩性病变
4. metabolic errors　　代谢异常
5. phenylketonuria　　苯丙酮尿症
6. Tay-Sachs diseases　　泰 - 萨克斯病
7. Niemann-Pick disease　　尼曼 - 克病
8. hypoglycemia　　低血糖症
9. hypocalcemia　　低钙血症
10. vitamin B_6 deficiency　　维生素 B_6 缺乏
11. inflammatory diseases　　炎性疾病
12. encephalitides　　脑炎
13. chronic alcoholism　　慢性酒精中毒
14. disturbance of cardiac rhythm　　心脏节律紊乱

II. Fill in the following blanks with one proper word.

Hardly any other illness can be traced back in medical history as far as epilepsy can. Many pointers from early history indicate that this (1) condition has been part of the human lot from the very beginning. Then as now, it is one of the most common chronic diseases and 0.5% of all human beings suffer from epilepsy, which means that in the U.K. alone around 300,000 to 600,000 people are (2) affected.

How can epilepsy be defined? When someone repeatedly has (3) epileptic seizures, then we say that that person is suffering from epilepsy. An epileptic seizure itself is one of the many pathological forms of reaction which can take place in the (4) brain; it is the brain's "response" or (5) reaction to a disturbing, irritating or damaging stimulus. This reaction to the stimulus is accompanied by abnormal electro-chemical excitatory processes in the (6) cerebral nerve cells. This pathological process takes place when suddenly an unnaturally large number of nerve cells are stimulated (7) simultaneously, causing a difference in voltage between the outer side of the cell wall and the inside of the cell (membrane potential). This voltage (8) difference is then suddenly discharged, creating a kind of "storm in the brain", or, to put it another way, "making a fuse blow".

If a person has one epileptic fit, it does not mean that he or she has epilepsy. Only when that person suffers (9) repeated spontaneous epileptic seizures (i.e. without any direct trigger), should he or she be diagnosed as having epilepsy. Epilepsy is therefore always a chronic illness which can go on for many years (but which does not necessarily last a lifetime!).

The term "epilepsy" is derived from the Greek word "epilambanein", which means "to seize upon", "to attack". Thus epilepsy is a (10) seizure or rather a disease which causes seizures to occur. As, however, there are many very different types of seizure, it is better to speak of epilepsies.

III. Write about 100 words describing the manifestations of epileptic seizures.

The most pronounced seizure is the generalized convulsion. The seizure itself begins with a cry preceding loss of consciousness and tonic stiffening of the body followed by clonic movements of all four extremities, the face, jaw, and head. Petit mal attacks are the minor seizures occurring in children, usually at a frequency of more than once a day and often as many as several hundred a day, with each attack lasting less than 1 minute. These seizures are characterized by a short staring episode, which may be associated with myoclonic jerks.

IV. Answer the following questions.

1. What is the difference between "epilepsy" and "seizures"?

   The term "epilepsy" merely means that the patient has seizures but does not connote the cause of the seizures.

2. What symptoms does a patient have if he/she suffers from generalized major motor seizure?

   Generalized major motor seizure begins with a cry preceding loss of consciousness and tonic stiffening of the body followed by clonic movements of all four extremities, the face, jaw, and head. *After seizure is a prolonged period of unconsciousness. During the attack, the patient may bite his tongue, experience urinary incontinence, and sustain injuries in a fall. The entire seizure lasts from 3 to 5 minutes and is followed by a period of coma or deep stupor. On arousing from the coma, the patient usually has a headache, and may vomit.*

3. What are the characteristics of petit mal attacks?

Petit mal attacks are the minor seizures occurring in children, usually at a frequency of more than one a day and often as many as several hundred a day, with each attack lasting less than 1 minute. These seizures are characterized by a short staring episode (petit mal absence), which may be associated with myoclonic jerks (myoclonic petit mal attacks). In some patients, the petit mal seizures are even shorter in duration and may consist of only a quick, sudden dropping of objects or falling to the floor (akinetic petit mal seizures), and these akinetic attacks may last only a fraction of a second.

4. Why is it said that laboratory studies are especially valuable to the diagnoses of a patient with epilepsy?

The answer is open.

Passage Three   Why We Forget

Exercises

I. Read the following statements and decide whether they are true or false. Then write T for true and F for false in the brackets.

[T] 1. When people suffer from memory loss, they usually think that they have got some serious brain disease.

[T] 2. It is implied that the Alzheimer disease is irreversible that will lead to memory loss.

[F] 3. The feelings of sadness and gloom that people sometimes have got in their daily life are the most common cause of intellectual deterioration.

[F] 4. Of the three ways to treat the clinical depression, electrotherapy is the most commonly applied and most effective.

[T] 5. Water present in the body plays an important role in adjusting the electrolyte concentrations.

[F] 6. The old people should be prescribed the same dosage of the medicine as the infants.

[T] 7. Alcohol abusers are predisposed to the loss of memory and other intellectual functions because they cannot get enough foods that contain vitamin B_{12}.

[T] 8. Hypoglycemia of the diabetics caused by too much insulin will change the patients' brain function and bring about memory problems.

[T] 9. Memory loss caused by head injury cannot be retrieved unless the brain damage is diagnosed and treated properly.

[F] 10. Excessive anti-hypertensive medicine leading to deficiency of blood supply to the brain will produce a loss of memory.

II. Here is a list of terms from the text. Analyze their meanings using the word building knowledge you have learned. Leave the space empty if the word part does not apply.

Term	Prefix	Root	Suffix	Chinese Translation
1. asymptomatic	a-	symptom	-atic	无症状的
2. antidepressant	anti-	depress	-ant	抗抑郁剂
3. malnutrition	mal-	nutri-	-tion	营养不良
4. geriatrics		gero-	-ics	老年病学
5. anemia	an-	-emia		贫血症

Chapter Six Skin

 Section A Medical Terminology

Learn the following combining forms, prefixes and suffixes for the skin and try to write in the blank space the literal meaning both in English and Chinese of the provided terminology.

Word Part	Meaning	Example Term	Meaning in English and Chinese
anthrac/o	coal 炭	anthracosis /ˌænθrəˈkəʊsɪs/	lung disease caused by the inhalation of coal dust 炭末沉着病
		anthracotherapy /ˌænθrəkəʊˈθerəpɪ/	treatment with charcoal 炭疗法
cutane/o, derm/o, dermat/o	skin 皮，皮肤	cutaneous /kjʊˈteɪnɪəs/	pertaining to the skin 皮肤的
		subcutaneous /ˌsʌbkjʊˈteɪnɪəs/	pertaining to beneath the skin 皮下的
		dermopathy /dɜːˈmɔːpəθɪ/	disease of the skin 皮肤病
		dermatology /dɜːməˈtɒlədʒɪ/	study of the skin 皮肤病学
diaphor/o	profuse sweating 多汗	diaphoresis /ˌdaɪəfəˈriːsɪs/	perspiration, especially profuse sweating 出汗
		diaphoretic /ˌdaɪəfəˈretɪk/	stimulating the secretion of sweat 发汗剂
-derma	skin 皮，皮肤	pyoderma /paɪəʊˈdɜːmə/	a purulent skin disease 脓皮病
		scleroderma /ˌsklɪrəˈdɜːmə/	hardening of the skin 硬皮病
hidr/o, sud/o	sweat 汗	hyperhidrosis /ˌhaɪpəhɪˈdrəʊsɪs/	excessive sweating 多汗症
		anhidrosis /ˌænhɪˈdrəʊsɪs/	condition characterized by little or no sweat production 无汗症
		sudorific /ˌsjuːdəˈrɪfɪk/	promoting the flow of sweat 发汗的，发汗药
		sudoresis /ˌsjuːdəˈriːsɪs/	excessive sweating 多汗
ichthy/o	scaly(fish-like) 鱼（鳞）的	ichthyosis /ˌɪkθɪˈəʊsɪs/	a dry, scaly condition of the skin 鱼鳞病
		ichthyotoxic /ɪkθaɪəʊˈtɒksɪk/	caused by the toxin from the fish 鱼毒的
kerat/o	horn 角质	keratosis /ˌkerəˈtəʊsɪs/	any horny growth（on the skin）角化病
		keratogenesis /ˌkerətəʊˈdʒenɪsɪs/	formation of the horny layer（of the skin）角质生成

Continue

Word Part	Meaning	Example Term	Meaning in English and Chinese
leuc/o leuk/o	white 白	leucocyte /ˈljuːkəsaɪt/	white blood cells 白细胞
		leukoderma /ljuːkəʊˈdɜːmə/	whitening of the skin 皮肤白斑病
melan/o	black 黑；black pigment 黑色素	melanoma /ˌmeləˈnəʊmə/	tumor of the black pigment cells 黑色素瘤
		melanocyte /ˈmelənəsaɪt/	cell that forms black pigment 黑素细胞
myc/o	fungus 真菌	dermatomycosis /ˌdɜːmətəʊmaɪˈkəʊsɪs/	fungal infection of the skin 皮真菌病，皮癣
		mycology /maɪˈkɒlədʒɪ/	study of the fungus 真菌学
onych/o	nail（指/趾）甲	onychomalacia /ˌɒnɪkəʊməˈleɪʃə/	softening of the nails 甲软化
		onychomycosis /ˌɒnɪkəʊmaɪˈkəʊsɪs/	fungal infection of the nail 甲癣
pil/o	hair 毛发；hair follicle 毛囊	piloerection /ˌpaɪləʊɪˈrekʃn/	hair standing on the end 立毛
		pilosebaceous /ˌpaɪləʊsɪˈbeɪʃəs/	pertaining to the hair follicle and sebaceous glands 毛囊皮脂的
seb/o	sebum 皮脂	seborrhea /sɪbɒˈrɪːə/	excessive secretion of sebum 皮脂溢
		sebaceous /sɪˈbeɪʃəs/	pertaining to the sebum 皮脂的
squam/o	scale-like 鳞状的	squamous /ˈskweɪməs/	pertaining to scale-like (cells) 鳞状的
		squamocellular /ˌskweɪməʊˈseljʊlə/	having squamous cells 鳞状细胞的
steat/o	fat 脂（肪）	steatoma /stiːəˈtəʊmə/	a sebaceous cyst 皮脂囊肿
		steatosis /ˌstiːəˈtəʊsɪs/	fatty degeneration 脂肪变性
trich/o	hair 毛，发	trichomycosis /trɪkəmaɪˈkəʊsɪs/	fungal infection of the hair 毛发菌病
		trichology /trɪˈkɒlədʒɪ/	study of the hair 毛发学
ungu/o	nail 指（趾）甲	ungula /ˈʌŋgjʊlə/	pertaining to the nail 指（趾）甲
		subungual /səbˈʌŋgjʊəl/	situated beneath a nail 甲下的
xanth/o	yellow 黄色	xanthoma /ˌzænˈθəʊmə/	tumor of yellow color 黄瘤
		xanthoderma /ˌzænθəʊˈdɜːmə/	yellowish discoloration of the skin 皮肤黄变

Exercises

Ⅰ. Match the anatomical terms in Column A with the correct definitions in Column B. Write the corresponding letter in the blank provided.

Column A	Column B
_D_ 1. melanocyte	A. excessive sweating
_E_ 2. epidermis	B. excessive secretion of sebum
_G_ 3. sebaceous gland	C. a tumor of yellow color in the skin
_F_ 4. sudoriferous gland	D. a cell that produces black pigment

B	5. seborrhea	E. the outer layer of the skin
C	6. xanthoma	F. sweat secreting gland of the skin
H	7. dermatoplasty	G. oil secreting gland of the skin
A	8. hyperhidrosis	H. surgical repair of the skin

II. Break down and define the word elements within each of the following terms, and then define the term itself.

Example:

cryosurgery	cryo/surgery	cold/surgery	cold surgery
1. anhidrosis	an/hidro/sis	without/sweat/condition	condition characterized by inadequate or no sweating
2. melanoma	melano/ma	black/tumor	black tumor (arising from melanocytes)
3. erythroderma	erythro/derma	red/skin	redness of the skin
4. seborrhea	sebo/rrhea	sebum/flow	excessive discharge of sebum
5. keratosis	kerato/sis	horn /condition	horny growth (on the skin)
6. sebaceous	seb/aceous	sebum/pertaining to	pertaining to sebum
7. subcutaneous	sub/cutane/ous	beneath/skin/pertaining to	pertaining to beneath the skin
8. transdermal	trans/derm/al	across/skin/pertaining to	pertaining to across the skin

III. Write a word for each of the following definitions.

1. condition characterized by little or no sweat production	anhidrosis
2. black pigment formed by melanocytes in epidermis	melanin
3. fungal infection of the nail	onychomycosis
4. perspiration, especially profuse sweating	diaphoresis
5. inflammation of the skin	dermatitis
6. the branch of medicine concerned with the hair and its diseases	trichology
7. yellow tumor (of the skin)	xanthoma
8. within the skin	intradermal

→ Section B   Reading Passages

Passage One   The Skin

Exercises

I. Match the word or expression in Column A with its description in Column B. Write the corresponding letter in the blank provided.

Column A	Column B
C 1. epidermis	A. The sac within which each hair grows
E 2. epithelium	B. Innermost layer of the skin, containing fat tissue

   A   3. hair follicle   C. The outermost layer of the skin

   D   4. mast cell   D. A cell found in connective tissue and in the corium layer of the skin. It secretes histamine and heparin

   B   5. subcutaneous tissue   E. The layer of skin cells forming the outer and inner surfaces of the body

   G   6. dermis   F. A gland that produces sebum, usually associated with a hair follicle

   H   7. keratin   G. The layer of the skin between the epidermis and the subcutaneous tissue

   F   8. sebaceous gland   H. A protein that thickens and toughens the skin and makes up hair and nails

   I   9. histamine   I. A substance released by mast cells in the corium during an allergic reaction

Ⅱ. Fill in the blanks in the following sentences with the proper terms given below. Change the form if necessary.

corium	melanocyte	fibroblast	melanin
lipocyte	histiocyte	hair follicle	basal layer

1. The cells that produce a dark pigment responsible for the coloration of hair and skin are called melanocytes.
2. A fat cell is known as a lipocyte.
3. A fiber-producing cell present in skin and connective tissues is called fibroblast.
4. A black pigment found in the epidermis is called melanin.
5. The deepest region of the epidermis is called the basal layer.
6. The hair follicle is a structure of the skin from which hair grows. It can be found all over the skin, with the exception of the lips, palms of the hands, and soles of the feet.
7. The middle layer of the skin is called the dermis or the corium.
8. A large phagocyte present in the connective tissue of the skin is called a histiocyte.

Ⅲ. Translate the following sentences into English.
1. 皮肤是脊椎动物的柔软覆盖物。
   Skin is the soft outer covering of vertebrates.
2. 在哺乳动物中，皮肤是皮肤系统 (integumentary system) 的一个器官。
   In mammals, the skin is an organ of the integumentary system.
3. 所有哺乳动物的皮肤上都有一些毛发，甚至看似无毛的海洋哺乳动物也有毛。
   All mammals have some hair on their skin, even marine mammals which appear to be hairless.
4. 皮肤与环境直接接触，是防御外来物入侵的第一道防线。
   The skin interfaces with the environment and is the first line of defense from external factors.
5. 皮肤具有保温、调节温度、感知等功能。
   The skin has functions of insulation, temperature regulation, sensation, and so on.

IV.Answer the following questions.

1. What are the three layers of the skin?

   The three layers of the skin are the epidermis, dermis, and subcutaneous tissue.

2. What are the accessory organs of the skin?

   The accessory organs of the skin are nails, hair, and the oil and sweat glands.

3. What are the functions of the skin and its accessory organs?

   The skin and its accessory organs help provide protection against injury, bacterial invasion, dehydration, and harmful ultraviolet rays. In addition, these structures play an important role in the regulation of body temperature and in the excretion of certain types of waste products formed in the body. The skin also contains many nerve endings and serves as a sensory receptor for pain, temperature, pressure, and touch.

4. In our daily life, especially in hot days, we can smell the special body odor of the people around us. Can you explain the phenomenon?

   The answer is open.

5. When you rub your skin as you take a bath, you will rub off some muddy dust from the skin. Does the thing that you rub off consist of only muddy dust? Why?

   The answer is open.

Passage Two   Disorders of the Skin

Exercises

I. Match each medical term in Column A with its description in Column B. Write the corresponding letter in the blank provided.

Column A		Column B
__C__	1. dermatology	A. an inflammatory disease of the sebaceous glands and hair follicles usually associated with excess secretion of sebum
__D__	2. Kaposi sarcoma	B. a defined discoloration of the skin; a congenital vascular tumor of the skin; a mole, birthmark
__A__	3. acne	C. a branch of medicine dealing with the skin and its diseases
__G__	4. comedo	D. cancerous lesion of the skin and other tissues seen most often in patients with AIDS
__H__	5. dermatitis	E. a fungus infection of the skin; ringworm
__E__	6. tinea	F. any skin condition marked by a thickened or horny growth
__F__	7. keratosis	G. a plug of sebum, often containing bacteria, in a hair follicle
__B__	8. nevus	H. inflammation of the skin, often associated with redness and itching which may be caused by allergy, irritants(contact dermatitis), or a variety of diseases
__I__	9. pruritus	I. severe itching

Ⅱ. Fill in the blanks with the correct terms of pathological skin conditions.

malignant melanoma	psoriasis	basal cell carcinoma
gangrene	squamous cell carcinoma	eczema
acne	tinea	scleroderma

1. malignant neoplasm originating in scale-like cells of the epidermis (squamous cell carcinoma)

2. a skin condition characterized by red pimples on the skin, especially on the face, due to inflamed or infected sebaceous glands and prevalent chiefly among adolescents (acne)

3. fungal skin infection (tinea)

4. chronic disease marked by hardening and shrinking of connective tissue in the skin (scleroderma)

5. necrosis of skin tissue resulting from ischemia (gangrene)

6. chronic or acute inflammatory skin disease with erythematous, pustular, or papular lesions (eczema)

7. cancerous tumor composed of melanocytes (malignant melanoma)

8. chronic, recurrent dermatosis marked by silvery gray scales covering red patches on the skin (psoriasis)

9. malignant neoplasm originating from the basal layer of the epidermis (basal cell carcinoma)

Ⅲ. Translate the following Chinese terms into English.

1. 痤疮   acne
2. 红斑   erythema
3. 湿疹   eczema
4. 坏疽   gangrene
5. 牛皮癣   psoriasis
6. 斑块   plaque
7. 鸡眼   corn
8. 芥子   mustard

Ⅳ. Discuss the following topics.

1. What are the symptoms of scleroderma?

   The symptom of scleroderma involves thickening and tightening of the skin. A very early sign of scleroderma is Raynaud disease, in which blood vessels in the fingers and toes constrict in the cold, causing numbness, pain, coldness, and tingling. Skin symptoms first appear on the forearms and around the mouth.

2. Which skin cancer tends not to metastasize?

   Squamous cell carcinoma.

3. Disorders of the skin are frequently seen in our life. What disorder did you see in yourself or in people around you? Please describe the symptoms.

   The answer is open.

Passage Three　Occupational Diseases of the Skin

Exercises

Ⅰ. Read the following statements and decide whether they are true or false. Then write T for true and F for false in the brackets.

[F] 1. People with an atopic body constitution are not easy to suffer from serious and lasting occupational contact dermatitis.

[T] 2. Cumulative insult dermatitis can result from one or more comparatively mild and marginal irritants.

[F] 3. Cellular components of the body are rarely damaged in a photoirritant reaction.

[F] 4. If the epidermal barrier has been fully reestablished, relapse may occur on relatively brief exposure to mild irritants.

[T] 5. The great majority of occupational contact dermatitis is associated with the hands along with other sites.

[F] 6. Irritant contact dermatitis can be easily tested clinically.

[F] 7. The symptomatic treatment of occupational contact dermatitis is different from that for any other types of dermatitis.

[T] 8. If a person with occupational contact dermatitis changes his disease-causing job, he may still have the dermatitis years later.

Ⅱ. Here is a list of terms from the text. Analyze their meanings using the word building knowledge you have learned. Leave the space empty if the word part does not apply.

Term	Prefix	Root	Suffix	Chinese Translation
1. dermatitis		dermato-	-itis	皮炎
2. erythema		erythro-	-ema	红斑
3. heterogeneous		hetero- gene	-ous	异源的
4. hyperpigmentation	hyper/	pigment-	-ation	色素沉着过度
5. hypopigmentation	hypo/	pigment-	-ation	色素减退
6. lymphocyte		lympho- -cyte		淋巴细胞
7. pathogenesis		patho- -gene	-sis	发病机制

Chapter Seven Oncology

→ Section A Medical Terminology

Learn the following combining forms, prefixes and suffixes pertaining to oncology and try to write in the blank space the literal meaning both in English and Chinese of the provided terminology.

Word Part	Meaning	Example Term	Meaning in English and Chinese
blast/o	embryonic 胚胎的；immature 未成熟的	neuroblastoma /ˌnjʊərəʊblæˈstəʊmə/	tumor of immature nerve tissue 成神经细胞瘤
		blastocyte /ˈblæstəʊˌsaɪt/	an embryonic cell 胚细胞
carcin/o	cancer 癌	carcinostatic /kaːsɪnəʊˈstætɪk/	stopping the growth of cancer 抑癌的
		carcinogenic /ˌkaːsɪnəˈdʒenɪk/	producing cancer 致癌的
-carcinoma	malignant tumor 恶性肿瘤，癌	adenocarcinoma /ˌædɪnəʊˌkaːsɪˈnəʊmə/	malignant tumor of a gland 腺癌
		hepatocarcinoma /ˌhepətəʊkaːsɪˈnəʊmə/	malignant tumor of liver 肝癌
cauter/o	burn 烧灼；腐蚀	cauterization /kɔːtəraɪˈzeɪʃən/	using burning to destroy tissues 烧灼术
		cauterant /ˈkɔːtərənt/	any burning or corrosive material 腐蚀剂；烧灼物
chem/o	chemical(s) 化学（物）	chemotherapy /ˌkiːməʊˈθerəpɪ/	using chemicals for (tumor) treatment 化疗
		chemocautery /keməʊˈkɔːtəri/	using chemicals to burn tissues 化学烙术
cry/o	cold 冷	cryosurgery /ˌkraɪəʊˈsɜːdʒərɪ/	using cold temperature to destroy tissue 冷冻手术
		cryogen /ˈkraɪəʊdʒən/	substance for producing low temperature 制冷剂
cyst/o	sac 囊；bladder 膀胱	cystoma /sɪsˈtəʊmə/	cystic tumor 囊瘤
		cystitis /sɪsˈtaɪtɪs/	inflammation of the bladder 膀胱炎

Continue

Word Part	Meaning	Example Term	Meaning in English and Chinese
epi-	upon, on 上；旁	epidermoid /ˌepɪ'dɜːrɪɔɪd/	resembling epidermal tissue 表皮样的
		epithelioma /epɪ,θiːlɪ'əʊmə/	an epithelial cancer 上皮癌
hist/o	tissue 组织	histogenesis /ˌhɪstəʊ'dʒenɪsɪs/	the formation of tissues 组织发生，组织生成
		histoblast /'hɪstəʊˌblæst/	immature tissue cell 成组织细胞
medull/o	bone marrow 骨髓；spinal cord 脊髓	medullary /'medələrɪ/	pertaining to the marrow 骨髓的；脊髓的
		medullitis /ˌmedə'laɪtɪs/	inflammation of the bone marrow or spinal cord 骨髓炎；脊髓炎
meta-	beyond 旁；change 转变	metastasis /mə'tæstəsɪs/	spread of a cancer beyond its original site to other areas（癌症）转移
		metamorphosis /ˌmetə'mɔːfəsɪs/	change of shape 变形
-oma	tumor 肿瘤	lymphoma /lɪm'fəʊmə/	tumor of lymph tissue 淋巴瘤
		dermatoma /dɜːmə'təʊmə/	tumor of skin 皮肤瘤
onc/o	tumor 肿瘤	oncology /ɒŋ'kɒlədʒɪ/	study of tumor 肿瘤学
		oncosis /ɒŋ'kəʊsɪs/	formation of tumor 肿瘤病
papill/o	nipple 乳头	papilloma /ˌpæpɪ'ləʊmə/	nipple like tumor 乳头状瘤
		papilliform /pæ'pɪlɪfɔːm/	in the form of a nipple 乳头状的
-plasia	formation 形成；growth 发育	hyperplasia /ˌhaɪpə'pleɪzɪə/	over development of an organ or tissue 增生
		dysplasia /dɪs'pleɪzɪə/	abnormal development 发育不良
-plasm	a growth, a formation 生成物	neoplasm /'niːəʊplæzəm/	a new growth 新生物，肿瘤
		nucleoplasm /'njʊklɪəˌplæzəm/	content inside the nucleus 核质
ple/o	many, more 多	pleomorphic /pliːə'mɔːfɪk/	having many shapes 多形的
		pleochromatic /ˌpliːəkrəʊ'mætɪk/	having many colors 多色的
radi/o	radiation 放射	radioscopy /ˌreɪdɪ'ɒskəpɪ/	using radiation for examination 放射检查
		radiotherapy /ˌreɪdɪəʊ'θerəpɪ/	treatment using radiation 放疗
-sarcoma	malignant connective tissue tumor 肉瘤	chondrosarcoma /ˌkɒndrəʊsɑː'kəʊmə/	malignant tumor of the cartilage 软骨肉瘤
		osteosarcoma /ˌɒstɪəʊsɑː'kəʊmə/	malignant tumor of the bone 骨肉瘤
scirrh/o	hard 硬；scirrhus 硬癌	scirrhous /'skɪrəs/	pertaining to scirrhus 硬癌的
		scirrhoma /skɪ'rəʊmə/	hard tumor 硬癌

Exercises

Ⅰ. Write the definitions of the following word parts.

1. meta-   <u>beyond; change</u>
2. papill/o   <u>nipple</u>
3. blast/o   <u>immature, enbryonic</u>
4. ple/o   <u>many; more</u>
5. cry/o   <u>cold</u>
6. onc/o   <u>tumor</u>
7. medull/o   <u>bone marrow, spinal cord</u>
8. cauter/o   <u>burn</u>
9. radi/o   <u>radiation</u>
10. chem/o   <u>chemical</u>

Ⅱ. Give the meaning of the following combining forms and try to figure out the meaning of each given word in Chinese.

1. carcin/o   <u>cancer</u>   carcinolysis   <u>癌细胞溶解</u>
2. cry/o   <u>cold</u>   cryoprobe   <u>冷冻探针</u>
3. hist/o   <u>tissue</u>   histology   <u>组织学</u>
4. onc/o   <u>tumor</u>   oncogene   <u>致癌基因</u>
5. -plasia   <u>growth</u>   hypoplasia   <u>发育不全</u>
6. -sarcoma   <u>malignant tumor</u> osteosarcoma   <u>骨肉瘤</u>
7. -plasm   <u>formation</u>   protoplasm   <u>原生质</u>
8. -oma   <u>tumor</u>   dermatoma   <u>皮肤瘤</u>

Ⅲ. Break down the following words and write their Chinese equivalents in the space given.

Example:

cytology   cyto/logy   细胞学
1. lipoma   <u>lip/oma</u>   脂肪瘤
2. cryosurgery   <u>cryo/surgery</u>   低温外科
3. fibroplasia   <u>fibro/plasia</u>   纤维组织形成
4. papillary   <u>papill/ary</u>   乳头的
5. carcinogenesis   <u>carcino/genesis</u>   致癌作用
6. osteoma   <u>oste/oma</u>   骨瘤
7. pleomastia   <u>pleo/mastia</u>   多乳房（畸形）
8. chondroblastoma <u>chondro/blast/oma</u>   成软骨细胞瘤
9. histoblast   <u>histo/blast</u>   成组织细胞
10. hemangiosarcoma <u>hem/angio/sarcoma</u>   血管肉瘤

Section B   Reading Passages

Passage One   Introduction to Cancer and Its Management

Exercises

Ⅰ. Fill in the following blanks with the terms in the box.

aberrant cell	melanoma
metastasize	asymptomatic
mutation	retinoblastoma
lymphoma	chromosome

1. A patient who exhibits no symptoms of disease is <u>asymptomatic</u>.
2. When tumor cells <u>metastasize</u>, the new tumor is called a secondary or metastatic tumor, and its cells are similar to those in the original tumor.
3. <u>Lymphoma</u> is cancer that begins in infection-fighting cells of the immune system, called lymphocytes.
4. In biology, a <u>mutation</u> is a permanent alteration of the nucleotide sequence of the genome of an organism, virus, or extrachromosomal DNA or other genetic elements.
5. <u>Melanoma</u> is a type of cancer that develops from the pigment-containing cells known as melanocytes.
6. At the molecular level, cancer is caused by mutation(s) in DNA, which result in <u>aberrant cell</u> proliferation.
7. A <u>chromosome</u> is a packaged and organized structure containing most of the DNA of a living organism.
8. <u>Retinoblastoma</u> is a rare form of cancer that rapidly develops from the immature cells of a retina, the light-detecting tissue of the eye.

Ⅱ. Read the following statements and decide whether they are true or false. Then write T for true and F for false in the brackets.

[F] 1. Cancers are destructive by the invasion of normal organs through direct and indirect extension to distant sites.
[T] 2. According to the passage, heart disease is expected to be surpassed by cancer as the most deadly disease in the 21st century.
[T] 3. A diet based on grains, vegetables, and fruits, is healthy to help prevent from having cancers.
[F] 4. The single most important carcinogen in the world is tobacco according to the passage.
[F] 5. Early detection is the best strategy to reduce cancer mortality because absolute prevention of cancer is not so realistic.

[F] 6. The diagnostic principle for cancer is to obtain adequate tissue from the tumor with few exceptions.

[F] 7. Biopsy might be a life-threatening procedure in the diagnosis of cancer.

[F] 8. Failure to detect a tumor that has extended to regional lymph nodes cannot lead to any under-treatment or any impression that the local treatment was not adequate.

Ⅲ.Translate the following sentences into English.

1. 癌症是第二大致命疾病，预计将很快超过心脏病而跃居恶性病首位。

Cancer is the second most deadly disease and is expected to surpass heart disease in a short time to top that nefarious list.

2. 约三分之一的癌症，特别是肺癌、食管癌和膀胱癌，是由吸烟引起或诱发的。

Smoking causes or contributes to the development of about one-third of all cancers, especially lung cancer, esophageal cancer and bladder cancer.

3. 如果由于缺乏有效措施而无法预防癌症的话，那么早期发现是降低癌症死亡率的最有效手段。

When prevention of cancer is not possible because effective means are lacking, early detection is the next best strategy to reduce cancer mortality.

4. 对于淋巴瘤来说，使用类固醇可能会出现肿瘤变小或症状缓解的情况。

As for a lymphoma, steroids may reduce the tumor size and relieve symptoms.

5. 医生不仅需要了解治疗措施，还需要了解自身的能力和局限性。

A doctor must know not only the therapeutic modalities, but also the skills and limitations of himself.

Ⅳ.Discuss the following topics.

1. What are the abnormal clinical behaviors of cancer cells?

   The abnormal clinical behaviors of cancer cells often consist of biologic aberrations such as genetic mutations, chromosomal translocations, expression of fetal or other discordant oncologic characteristics, and the inappropriate secretion of hormones or enzymes.

2. What are the main agents that will lead to the development of cancer?

   Promoters and suppressors play a central role of developing cancer in many cases. Chemicals such as benzene and nitrosamines, physical agents such as gamma and ultraviolet radiation, and biologic agents such as the Epstein--Barr and hepatitis viruses contribute to carcinogenesis under certain circumstances. Dietary factors, inherited susceptibilities, Down syndrome and the Li-Fraumeni syndrome all are harbingers of a substantial risk for developing various cancers.

3. What are the main diagnostic principles and therapeutic principles for cancer?

   The first diagnostic principle is that adequate tissue must be obtained from the tumor to establish the specific diagnosis and subtype of cancer. A second diagnostic principle is to establish the extent of the disease.

   The first step in treatment is to know the patient. The second step is to know the tumor.

Third, one must know the available therapies. Finally, one must know oneself: one's skills, experience, objectivity, and limitations.

4. What should a doctor pay attention to when he treats a patient with cancer?

The answer is open.

Passage Two   Characteristics of Benign and Malignant Neoplasms

Exercises

I. Sum up the characteristics of benign and malignant tumors and write them in the following table.

Characteristics	Benign Tumors	Malignant Tumors
differentiation and anaplasia	well specialized/differentiated cells	a wide range of parenchymal cell differentiation, from surprisingly well-differentiated to completely undifferentiated
rate of growth	grow slowly	multiply rapidly
local invasion	localized at its site of origin, characteristically encapsulated and not invasive and infiltrative	characteristically invasive and infiltrative and no well-defined capsules
metastasis	not spread to form secondary tumor masses in other places	spread to form secondary tumor masses in other places

II. Fill in the following blanks with the terms in the box. Change the form if necessary.

proliferation	menopause	leukemia	glycogen
promoter	susceptibility	metastasis	Down syndrome

1. Menopause is defined as the absence of menstrual periods for 12 months. It is the time in a woman's life when the function of the ovaries ceases.
2. Leukemia is a group of cancers that usually begin in the bone marrow and result in high numbers of abnormal white blood cells.
3. A complex material made of individual glucose molecules, mainly stored in the liver and muscle cells is called glycogen.
4. In genetics, a promoter is a region of DNA that initiates transcription of a particular gene.
5. Identifying the genes involved in susceptibility to cancer may have potential utility in risk management and lead to greater understanding of the biological pathways involved in cancer development.
6. Proliferation is a rapid multiplication of parts or the increase in the number of cells.
7. Down syndrome occurs when an individual has a full or partial extra copy of chromosome 21.
8. The process by which cancer spreads from the place at which it first arose as a primary tumor to distant locations in the body is called metastasis.

Ⅲ.Write a word for each of the following definitions.

1. Loss of structural differentiation, especially as seen in malignant neoplasms ____anaplasia____

2. Development of fibrous tissue in the stromal cells ____stromal fibrosis____

3. An abnormal growth of tissue caused by the rapid division of cells that have undergone some form of mutation ____neoplasm____

4. A hard slow-growing malignant tumor having a preponderance of fibrous tissue ____scirrhous tumor____

5. Primary tissue that constitutes the essential part of an organ ____parenchyma____

6. The ordinary process of cell division ____mitosis____

7. The process of a cell changing from one cell type to another ____cellular differentiation____

8. Marked variation in size and shape ____pleomorphism____

9. A complex of DNA and proteins that forms chromosomes within the nucleus of eukaryotic cells ____chromatin____

10. Benign smooth muscle tumors ____leiomyomas____

Ⅳ.Fill in each blank with one proper word.

The word tumor is a broad term to identify any (1) growth within the body but has become synonymous with a benign or malignant growth. At times the word neoplasm is used which is essentially a new growth of (2) tissue that has no purpose or function in the body.

A tumor arises from uncontrolled or an (3) abnormal growth of cells that has no physiological function in the body, occupies space or destroys surrounding tissue to fit in the specific area and can affect the (4) function or health of the organ it affects.

Tumors should not be confused with other growth phenomena in the body like hyperplasia or hypertrophy. These terms are used when an (5) organ enlarges or when there is an increase in the organ's cells or layers of tissue than would be considered the norm leading to an increase in size of the affected organ. This (6) enlargement is not a tumor.

Simply, there are two types of tumors — (7) benign or (8) malignant. A benign tumor is not always thought of in the same serious light as malignant tumors. Benign growths usually have little or no (9) clinical effect; however, depending on the location, a benign tumor can cause a number of signs or symptoms if it presses against important neighboring organs like a gland or nerve. A malignant tumor invades the surrounding tissue while growing in (10) size, destroying organs and tissue and may spread to other areas of the body.

Passage Three My experience of malignant melanoma

Exercises

Ⅰ. Read the following statements and decide whether they are true or false. Then write T for true and F for false in the brackets.

[F] 1. When the author receives a cancer diagnosis, she still couldn't imagine it could fall on her.

[T] 2. The author felt surprised and poignant when being told she had a malignant melanoma, because she had been a dermatology nurse for many years.

[F] 3. Melanocytes, which are found in the basal layer of the epidermis, always do harm to our body.

[F] 4. Most of melanomas start from an existing mole or freckle, without any change of normal color.

[T] 5. According to the story, the author experienced three surgeries.

[F] 6. After receiving the report, the author was relieved that the tumor was shallow and had been completely removed with the first excision without any worry.

[T] 7. The author had been struggling to accept the fact that the skin color of her leg's appearance has changed forever.

[F] 8. According to the author, she couldn't have any awareness in the areas of the wound.

[F] 9. Although the grafted area was very tender, the author still used tight stockings after the surgery to help minimize postoperative swelling of her lower leg.

[T] 10. The author removed the primary dressing and applied a silicone-based product.

II. Here is a list of terms from the text. Analyze their meanings using the word building knowledge you have learned. Leave the space empty if the word part does not apply.

Term	Prefix	Root	Suffix	Chinese Translation
1. melanoma		melan/o	-oma	黑色素瘤
2. melanocyte		melan/o -cyte		黑素细胞
3. epidermis	epi-	dermis		上皮, 表皮
4. hypersensitivity	hyper-	sensitivity		过敏症
5. micrometastasis	micro-	metastasis		微小转移

Section A Medical Terminology

Learn the following combining forms, prefixes and suffixes related to drugs and try to write in the blank space the literal meaning both in English and Chinese of the provided terminology.

Word Part	Meaning	Example Term	Meaning in English and Chinese
aer/o	air or gas 气	aerogenic /ˌeərəʊˈdʒenɪk/	producing gas 产气的
		aerotonometer /ˌeərəʊtəˈnɒmɪtə/	an instrument for measuring the pressure of the gas 气体张力计
anti-	against 对抗	antidiuretic /ˌæntɪˌdaɪjʊəˈretɪk/	an agent that acts against urination 抗利尿药
		antihypertensive /ˌæntɪˌhaɪpəˈtensɪv/	an agent that acts against hypertension 抗高血压药
algesi/o	pain 痛	algesic /ælˈdʒesɪk/	relating to pain 疼痛的
		analgesic /ˌænəlˈdʒiːzɪk/	an agent that relieves pain 止痛剂
bacteri/o	bacterium (pl. *bacteria*) 细菌	bacteriemia /ˌbæktɪəˈriːmɪə/	presence of bacteria in blood 菌血症
		antibacterial /ˌæntɪbækˈtɪərɪəl/	acting against bacteria 抗菌的
coagul/o	clotting 凝块	anticoagulant /ˌæntɪkəʊˈægjʊlənt/	an agent that prevents blood clotting 抗凝剂
		coagulation /kəʊˈægjʊleɪʃən/	clotting 凝结
erg/o	work 工作；力	synergy /ˈsɪnədʒɪ/	combined actions, as of drugs 协同作用
		ergogenic /ɜːgəʊˈdʒenɪk/	producing work output 功能增进的
esthesi/o	feeling, sensation 感觉	anesthesia /ˌænəsˈθiːʒə/	loss of sensation 麻醉
		anesthesiology /ˌænɪsˌθiːziːˈɒlədʒɪ/	study of anesthesia and anesthetics 麻醉学
fung/o	fungus 真菌	fungicide /ˈfʌndʒɪˌsaɪd/	an agent that kills fungus 杀真菌剂
		antifungal /ˌæntɪˈfʌŋgəl/	acting against fungus 抗真菌的

Continue

Word Part	Meaning	Example Term	Meaning in English and Chinese
-gen	origin, producer 源头，原	antigen /'æntɪdʒən/	producer of defense 抗原
		pathogen /'pæθədʒən/	origin of disease 病原
hypn/o	sleep 睡；hypnosis 催眠	hypnogenic /ˌhɪpnəʊ'dʒenɪk/	inducing sleep 催眠的
		hypnotherapy /ˌhɪpnəʊ'θerəpɪ/	using hypnosis for treatment 催眠疗法
-lytic	destroying or dissolving 溶解	hepatolytic /ˌhepətəʊ'lɪtɪk/	destroying the liver cells 溶解肝细胞的
		thrombolytic /ˌθrɒmbəʊ'lɪtɪk/	dissolving a thrombus 溶解血栓的
narc/o	stupor 昏迷	narcosis /naː'kəʊsɪs/	in a state of stupor 昏迷状态
		narcotic /naː'kɒtɪk/	an agent that produces stupor 镇静剂
pharmac/o	drug 药	pharmacometrics /ˌfaːməkəʊ'metrɪks/	measurement of the drugs 药物测量学
		pharmacology /ˌfaːmə'kɒlədʒɪ/	study of drugs 药学
prurit/o	itching 痒	antipruritic /ˌæntɪprʊ'rɪtɪk/	an agent that relieves itching 止痒剂
		pruritogenic /ˌprʊrɪtəʊ'dʒenɪk/	producing itch 引起瘙痒的
py/o	pus 脓	antipyogenic /ˌæntɪpaɪəʊ'dʒenɪk/	preventing the development of pus 防止化脓的
		pyorrhea /ˌpaɪəʊ'riːə/	flow of pus 溢脓
pyret/o	fever 发热	antipyretic /ˌæntɪpaɪ'retɪk/	an agent that relieves fever 退热剂
		pyretogen /paɪə'retədʒen/	a substance that causes fever 热原，致热物
pyr/o, pyrot/o	fire 火；heat 热	antipyrotic /æntɪpaɪ'rɒtɪk/	an agent that treats burns 治灼伤药
		pyrogen /'paɪərədʒən/	a heat producing substance 热原质
-static	inhibiting 抑制；inhibiting agent 抑制剂	bacteriostatic /bækˌtɪərɪə'stætɪk/	an agent that inhibits the growth of bacteria 抑菌剂
		fungistatic /'fʌndʒɪˌstætɪk/	an agent that inhibits the growth of fungus 抑真菌剂
toxic/o	toxin, poison 毒	toxicemia /tɒksɪ'siːmɪə/	presence of toxin in blood 毒血症
		toxicology /tɒksɪ'kɒlədʒɪ/	study of the toxin 毒理学
vir/o	virus 病毒	viricide /'vaɪrɪsaɪd/	an agent that kills viruses 杀病毒剂
		virosis /vaɪ'rəʊsɪs/	viral disease 病毒病

Exercises

Ⅰ. Write the definitions of the following combining forms, prefixes and suffixes and then provide an example word for each of them.

1. coagul/o   clotting   anticoagulant
2. pyret/o   fever   antipyretic
3. fung/o   mold, fungus   fungicide
4. narc/o   stupor   narcosis
5. vir/o   virus   antiviral
6. hypn/o   sleep   hypnogenic
7. -lytic   destroying or dissolving   thrombolytic
8. prurit/o   itching   antipruritic
9. pyr/o   fire, heat   antipyrotic
10. vir/o   virus   viremia

Ⅱ. Define the following drug classification terms. Where possible, break the word down into its word elements such as prefix, word root, combining vowel and suffix in the space provided.

Prefix	Combining Form	Suffix

1. analgesic

an agent that relieves pain without causing loss of consciousness

| an | / | alges | / | ic |

2. antiarrhythmic

an agent that controls cardiac arrhythmias

| anti | / | arrhythm | / | ic |

3. antihistamine

an agent that blocks the action of histamine and relieves the allergic symptoms

| anti | / | hist | / | amine |

4. antipyretic

an agent that relieves or reduces fever

| anti | / | pyret | / | ic |

5. antineoplastic

an agent that prevents the growth of neoplastic cells

| anti | / | neo/plast | / | ic |

6. anticoagulant

an agent that prevents blood clotting

| anti | / | coagul | / | ant |

7. antipyrotic

an agent that is effective in the treatment of burns

| anti | / | pyrot | / | ic |

8. antipruritic

   an agent that relieves or reduces itching

   | anti | / | prurit | / | ic |

9. antibiotic

   an agent that inhibits or kills germ life

   | anti | / | bi/o | / | tic |

10. antifungal

    an agent that destroys or inhibits the growth of fungi

    | anti | / | fung | / | al |

III. Match each word part in Column A with its English term in Column B. Write the corresponding letter in the blank provided.

Column A		**Column B**
C	1. algi/o	A. air
E	2. esthesi/o	B. work
G	3. narc/o	C. pain
B	4. erg/o	D. destroying
D	5. -lytic	E. feeling
A	6. aer/o	F. fungus
F	7. myc/o	G. stupor
J	8. vir/o	H. origin, producer
I	9. pharmac/o	I. drug
H	10. -gen	J. virus

→ **Section B   Reading Passages**

Passage One   Drugs

Exercises

I. Complete the following sentences with the words or phrases given below.

drug action	toxicologist	chemical	generic or official
trade or brand	potentiation	antineoplastic	pharmacologist

1. The name that describes the chemical structure of a drug is the <u>chemical</u> name.

2. The name of a drug that is established when the drug is first manufactured is known as the <u>generic or official</u> name.

3. The name by which a drug is sold by a specific manufacturer is known as the <u>trade or brand</u> name.

4. A person specializing in the study of the harmful effects of drugs on the body is a <u>toxicologist</u>.

5. How the drug produces changes within the body is known as <u>drug action</u>.

6. A person (often a medical doctor) who specializes in the study of the actions of drugs is known as a <u>pharmacologist</u>.

7. <u>Potentiation</u> is another term for synergism.

8. <u>Antineoplastic</u> agents act to destroy cancer cells.

II. Using the drug classifications below, write the most appropriate response in the space provided.

antiulcer agent	antitussive	antianginal	anticonvulsant	diuretic
antacid	antihistamine	anesthetic	antibiotic	antidiabetic
antihypertensive	antiemetic	anticoagulant	antidepressant	analgesic

1. Juan Miguel is complaining of a headache. His doctor told him to take Tylenol (acetaminophen) to relieve the pain.

   That acetaminophen is classified as an <u>analgesic</u>.

2. Judy Silverstein's mother recently died shortly after Judy lost her job. For the last two months Judy has been having difficulty coping with her situation. She has been extremely depressed and cried excessively. The doctor has placed Judy on Elavil (amitriptyline hydrochloride), a medication used to alleviate mental depression.

   That amitriptyline hydrochloride is classified as an <u>antidepressant</u>.

3. Latasha Smith has had a cold for three days. She has developed a scratchy cough that keeps her awake at night. Her doctor recommended that she purchase Robitussin PE (pseudoephedrine hydrochloride and guaifenesin) at her local pharmacy.

   That pseudoephedrine hydrochloride and guaifenesin is classified as an <u>antitussive</u>.

4. Pearl Henderson suffers from high blood pressure. The doctor has placed her on Corgard (nadalol), a medication used to control hypertension.

   That nadolol is classified as an <u>antihypertensive</u>.

5. Bette Daves was stung by a wasp while working in her garden. Shortly after the sting, her finger was throbbing and she noticed some swelling. She immediately took one of her Benadryl capsules (diphenhydramine hydrochloride) to relieve the allergic response to the sting.

   That diphenhydramine hydrochloride is classified as an <u>antihistamine</u>.

6. Mark Jones has an ear infection. His pediatrician has prescribed Bactrim (trimethoprim and sulfamethoxazole) to stop the infection.

   That trimethoprim and sulfamethoxazole is classified as an <u>antibiotic</u>.

7. Helen Bell has experienced a good bit of swelling in her legs lately. Her physician has prescribed Lasix (furosemide), a medication used to increase urine secretion, in hopes of

relieving the edema in her legs.

That furosemide is classified as a <u>diuretic</u>.

8. Priscilla Conner is 4 months pregnant and is still complaining of nausea. Her physician has prescribed Bonine (meclizine hydrochloride) to relieve the nausea.

That meclizine hydrochloride is classified as an <u>antiemetic</u>.

9. Tony Tangorre went to the dentist today to have a filling replaced. His dentist used Xylocaine (lidocaine) to completely numb the tooth before replacing the filling.

That lidocaine is classified as an <u>anesthetic</u>.

Ⅲ.Translate the following sentences into English.

1. 最好饭后服用本药。

The medicine should be administered after meals preferably.

2. 本药对中枢神经系统有兴奋作用。

This drug exerts a stimulant effect on the central nervous system.

3. 副作用是因常规用药而引起的毒性作用。

Side effects are toxic effects that routinely result from the use of a drug.

4. 舌下给药一片后，20～30 秒内即可起到缓解作用。

Sublingual administration of one tablet acts within 20~30 seconds with soothing effects.

5. 维生素不仅可以从蔬菜中摄取，还可以在体内合成。

Vitamins are not only taken up from vegetable sources but also synthesized in the body.

Ⅳ.Discuss the following topics.

1. What are the three different names of a drug? Please describe them briefly.

   A drug can have three different names. The chemical name is the chemical formula for the drug. This name is often long and complicated. The generic or official name is a shorter, less complicated name that is recognized as identifying the drug for legal and scientific purposes. The brand name or trade name is the private property of the individual drug manufacturer, and no competitor may use it. Brand names often have the superscript ® after or before the name indicating that this is a registered trade name.

2. How many routes of drug administration are mentioned in the passage? What are the advantages and disadvantages of each route of drug administration in your opinion?

   The answer is open.

3. What is drug action? Please describe the five terms concerning the action and interaction of drugs in your own words.

   The answer is open.

4. Drug toxicity is the poisonous and potentially dangerous effects of some drugs. In your opinion, how should physicians be trained to be competent and be aware of the potential toxic effects of all drugs they prescribe?

   The answer is open.

Passage Two   Prescription and Over-the-counter Drugs

Exercises

Ⅰ. Match the abbreviations in Column A with the appropriate definitions in Column B. Write the corresponding letter in the blank provided.

	Column A		Column B
F	1. a.c.	A.	milligram
E	2. b.i.d.	B.	freely, as needed
G	3. cap(s).	C.	as directed
K	4. sig.	D.	four times a day
J	5. gtt.	E.	twice a day
I	6. p.o.	F.	before meals
C	7. u.d.	G.	capsule
H	8. h.s.	H.	at bedtime
L	9. t.i.d.	I.	orally
B	10. ad lib.	J.	drop
A	11. mg.	K.	write on label
M	12. q.4.h.	L.	three times a day
D	13. q.i.d.	M.	every 4 hours

Ⅱ. Translate the following sentences into English.

1. 处方药只能由医生处方开出。

Prescription drugs can be ordered and prescribed only by a physician.

2. 当使用或服用药物时，病人应了解该药物的副作用。

When consumers use or take medications, they should acquaint themselves with their side effects.

3. 非处方药指的是不用处方就能买到的药。

OTC drugs are those products available without prescription.

4. 购买非处方药前，必须确定是否真正需要此药。

Before purchasing an OTC drug, one should be certain that the substance is actually needed.

5. 若症状持续超过 24 小时，请看医生。

If symptoms persist more than 24 hours, go to see your doctor.

Ⅲ. Fill in the blanks with one proper word.

Over-the-counter (OTC) medicines are drugs you can buy without a prescription. Some OTC medicines relieve aches, pains and itches. Some prevent or (1) cure diseases, like tooth decay and athlete's foot. Others help manage recurring problems, like migraines. In the United States, the Food and Drug Administration decides whether a medicine is (2) safe enough to sell over-the-counter. Taking OTC medicines still has risks. Some (3) interact with other medicines, supplements, foods or drinks. Others (4) <u>cause</u> problems for people with certain medical conditions. If you're pregnant, talk to your healthcare provider before (5) <u>taking</u> any medicines.

It is important to take medicines correctly, and be careful when giving them to children. More medicine does not (6) <u>necessarily</u> mean better. You should never take OTC medicines longer or in higher (7) <u>doses</u> than the label recommends. If your symptoms don't go away, it's a clear (8) <u>signal</u> that it's time to see your healthcare provider.

Ⅳ.Discuss the following topics.

1. What are the basic types of drugs and their synonyms on the market?

   There are two basic types of drugs, or medicines, prescription (R) and over-the-counter (OTC) drugs. Prescription drugs are also referred to as legend drugs. OTC substances may also be referred to as proprietary, ethical proprietary, patent, and home medicines.

2. What should an individual consider when he plans to use prescription drugs?

   He should be familiar with the prescription labels, which should contain the following information: individual's name, physician's name, pharmacy name, address, telephone number, name of the medication (if the physician tells the pharmacist to include it), how often and when to take the medication, how much to take each time and any special instructions for use.

3. Illustrate the contents of a physician's prescription and list some of the common symbols found thereon.

   The answer is open.

Passage Three　Human Immunodeficiency Virus (HIV) Screening Test

Exercises

Ⅰ. Read the following statements and decide whether they are true or false. Then write T for true and F for false in the brackets.

[T] 1.　The HIV peptides are immobilized on the membrane of the test cassette.

[F] 2.　The peptides on the membrane of the cassette are practically non-infectious and are extremely specific for HIV antibody detection.

[T] 3.　AIDS is transmitted by sexual contact, exposure to blood or certain blood products, and from an infected mother to her fetus or child through childbirth or breast-feeding.

[F] 4.　Only darker test dots indicate positive results.

[F] 5.　In the test kit, there are only two dropper bottles and one cassette.

[T] 6.　It is suggested that all human source specimens be treated cautiously, as they are likely to be infectious.

[T] 7.　Before the test is performed, all reagents and specimens must be brought to room temperature.

[F] 8.　The HIV screening test is designed for use with whole blood only; serum and plasma are not supposed to be used.

[F] 9.   Background pink color present at the end of the test indicates a negative result.

[T] 10. If the test result is positive, a confirmatory test should be run.

Ⅱ. Here is a list of terms from the text. Analyze their meanings using the word building knowledge you have learned. Leave the space empty if the word part does not apply.

Term	Prefix	Root	Suffix	Chinese Translation
1. antibody	anti-	body		抗体
2. recombinant	re-	combin-	-ant	重组
3. microbiological	micro-	biologi-	-cal	微生物学的
4. biomedical	bio-	medi-	-cal	生物医学的
5. disinfectant	dis-	infect	-ant	消毒剂
6. glycoprotein		glyco- protein		糖蛋白

Chapter Nine High-Tech Medicine

 Section A   Medical Terminology

Learn the following combining forms, prefixes and suffixes and try to write in the blank space the literal meaning both in English and Chinese of the provided terminology.

Word Part	Meaning	Example Term	Meaning
ambi-	both 双，两	ambilateral /ˌæmbɪˈlætərəl/	bilateral, of two sides 两侧的
		ambiopia /ˌæmbɪˈəʊpɪə/	double vision 复视
-apheresis	removal 分离	lymphocytapheresis /ˌlɪmfəʊˌsaɪtəfəˈriːsɪs/	removal of lymph cells in blood 淋巴细胞分离术
		plasmapheresis /ˌplæzməfəˈriːsɪs/	removal of plasma from blood 血浆分离术
geno-	produce 生成；gene 基因	genotype /ˈdʒenətaɪp/	genetic constitution of an individual 基因型
		genotoxic /dʒɪnəˈtɒksɪk/	damaging to genes 基因毒性的
-gel	glue 胶；colloid 凝胶	aerogel /ˈeərədʒel/	colloid containing gas 气凝胶
		silicagel /ˈsɪlɪkədʒel/	colloid made from silica 硅胶
iatr/o	treatment 治疗	iatrogenic /ˌaɪətrəʊˈdʒenɪk/	caused by treatment 医源性的
		psychiatry /saɪˈkaɪətrɪ/	treatment of mental illness 精神病学
-ics	discipline 学，学科	metabolomics /mɪtæˌbəˈlɒmɪks/	study of the metabolism 代谢学
		proteomics /ˌprəʊtɪˈɒmɪks/	study of proteomes and their functions 蛋白组学
iso-	same 同	isotope /ˈaɪsətəʊp/	atoms with the same atomic number 同位素
		isotype /ˈaɪsəʊtaɪp/	of the same type 同形
neo-	new 新	neonatal /niːəʊˈneɪtəl/	new born 新生儿
		neocortex /niːəʊˈkɒteks/	new cortex 新皮层
-ome	complete set 组	proteome /ˈprəʊtɪəʊm/	complete set of proteins (in an organism) 蛋白组
		genome /ˈdʒiːnəʊm/	complete set of genes (in an organism) 基因组

Continue

Word Part	Meaning	Example Term	Meaning
-on	a small particle 粒子; substance 元素	interferon /ˌɪntəˈfɪərɒn/	a substance that interferes (the duplication of virus) 干扰素
		electron /ɪˈlektrɒn/	a negatively charged particle 电子
para-	at the side of, beside 旁，副	paracentral /ˈpærɪsentrəl/	near a center 旁中央的
		paracardiac /pærəˈkɑːdɪæk/	beside the heart 心旁的
-poiesis	formation 生成	erythropoiesis/ /ɪˌrɪθrəʊpɒɪˈiːsɪs/	formation of red blood cells 红细胞生成
		cytopoiesis /ˌsaɪtəʊpɒɪˈiːsɪs/	formation of cells 细胞生成
-poietin	a substance that stimulates the formation (of cells) 生成素	angiopoietin /ˌændʒɪəʊpɒɪˈiːtɪn/	a substance that stimulates the formation of vessels 血管生成素
		erythropoietin /ɪˌrɪθrəʊpɒɪˈiːtɪn/	a substance that stimulates the formation of red blood cells 红细胞生成素
poly-, pluri-	many, much 多	polyneuropathy /pɒlɪnjʊəˈrɒpəθɪ/	disease affecting many nerves 多神经病
		polymyositis /pɒlɪmaɪəˈsaɪtɪs/	inflammation affecting many muscles 多肌炎
		pluripotent /ˌpluəriˈpəʊtənt/	capable of differentiating into different types of cell 多能的
		plurinuclear /ˌpluəriˈnjuːklɪə/	having many nuclei 多核的
stere/o-	solid 实体; three dimensional 三维的	stereoanesthesia /ˌsterɪəʊˈnesθiːzɪə/	reduced ability to identify objects 实体觉缺失
		stereomicroscope /ˌsterɪəʊˈmaɪkrəskəʊp/	a microscope to view three dimensional objects 立体显微镜
steth/o-	chest 胸	stethomyitis /steθəʊmɪˈaɪtɪs/	inflammation of the muscles of the chest 胸肌炎
		stethoscope /ˈsteθəskəʊp/	an instrument to hear the sound from the chest 听诊器
-taxis	arrangement 位置; direction of movement 趋向	stereotaxis /ˌsterɪəʊˈtæksɪs/	movement of an organism in response to the stimulus of a solid object 趋实体性
		phototaxis /ˌfəʊtəʊˈtæksɪs/	movement of an organism in response to light 趋光性
ultra-	beyond 超，高倍	ultramicroscope /ˌʌltrəˈmaɪkrəskəʊp/	an instrument to view beyond ordinary microscope 超高倍显微镜
		ultrasonography /ˌʌltrəsəˈnɒgrəfɪ/	process of recording with ultrasound 超声波扫描术
vers/i	turning 转	reversible /rɪˈvɜːsɪbəl/	able to turn back 可逆的
		introversion /ˌɪntrəʊˈvɜːʃn/	turning inward 内向性

Exercises

Ⅰ. Fill in the following blanks with the terms in the box.

leukopoiesis	polyneuropathy
genotoxicity	metabolomics
ultrasonography	stethoscope
chemotaxis	genome

1. The formation of the white blood cells are called <u>leukopoiesis</u>.

2. The <u>stethoscope</u> is an acoustic medical device for auscultation, or listening to the internal sounds of an animal or human body.

3. In genetics, <u>genotoxicity</u> describes the property of chemical agents that is toxic to the genetic information within a cell, which may lead to mutations.

4. <u>Ultrasonography</u> uses high-frequency sound (ultrasound) waves to produce images of internal organs and other tissues.

5. A <u>genome</u> is an organism's complete set of DNA, including all of its genes.

6. The movement of an organism or cell in response to a chemical stimulus is called <u>chemotaxis</u>.

7. <u>Polyneuropathy</u> is the simultaneous malfunction of many peripheral nerves throughout the body.

8. <u>Metabolomics</u> is the scientific study of chemical processes involved in metabolism.

Ⅱ. Write the English and Chinese meanings of the following term.

1. pediatrics   <u>the treatment of children's illness 儿科学</u>
2. ambisexual   <u>pertaining to both sexes 两性的</u>
3. neutron   <u>a particle that carries no electric charge 中子</u>
4. dynamics   <u>the study of the forces that causes movement 动力学</u>
5. irreversible   <u>unable to be turned back 不可逆的</u>
6. ultrafilter   <u>a filter that separates very fine particles 超滤器</u>
7. isomorphic   <u>having the same shape 同形状的</u>
8. leukopoietin   <u>a substance that stimulates the formation of the white blood cells 白细胞生成素</u>

Ⅲ. Match the combining form, prefix and suffix in Column A with its definition in Column B. Write the corresponding letter in the blank provided.

Column A	Column B
<u>C</u> 1. ultra-	A. many, much
<u>G</u> 2. ambi-	B. arrangement, direction of movement
<u>A</u> 3. poly-, pluri-	C. beyond
<u>E</u> 4. iso-	D. discipline
<u>B</u> 5. -taxis	E. same
<u>H</u> 6. -ome	F. formation
<u>D</u> 7. -ics	G. both

F	8. -poiesis	H. complete set
J	9. vers/i	.I. gene
I	10. gen/o	J. turning

→ Section B Reading Passages

Passage One A New Initiative on Precision Medicine

Exercises

I. Match the technologies in Column A with their descriptions in Column B.

Column A	Column B
J 1. anti-bleeding gel	A. It is a method by which an object is suspended with no support other than magnetic fields. Magnetic force is used to counteract the effects of the gravitational acceleration and any other accelerations.
A 2. magnetic levitation	B. Developed by a Canadian researcher, it delivers a small electrical charge every ten minutes. The effect is the same as if the patient was moving on their own — it activates muscles and increases circulation in that area, and effectively eliminates bed sores, thereby saving lives.
C 3. artificial cell mimicry	C. The material is formed in bunches that are only 7.5 billionths of a meter wide — for comparison, that's about four times wider than a DNA double helix. Cells have their own type of skeleton, known as a cytoskeleton, which is made of proteins. The synthetic gel will take the place of that cytoskeleton in a cell, and when it's applied to, say, a wound, it replaces any cells that were lost or damaged.
D 4. brain cells from urine	D. The method uses ordinary cells present in urine, and transforms them into neural progenitor cells — the precursors of brain cells.
B 5. electric underwear	E. The pollen is used as means to provide life-saving vaccines. The allergens are removed from the pollen, and a vaccine is then injected into the empty space left behind. Research like this could vastly change the way vaccines and medications can be given to human.

   E   6. pollen vaccines

   F. Using 3D printers, researchers have developed a hybrid material that has the same properties — the same strength and flexibility — as a real bone.

   F   7. printed bones

   G. DNA building blocks have been pieced together to form a multitude of Lego-like bricks by researchers at Harvard University and Massachusetts Institute of Technology in the US. The bricks are nanoscopic, but can be locked together like children's Lego blocks and have been used to create more than one hundred distinct shapes with complex surfaces, as well interiors with pores and tunnels.

   H   8. brain damage repair

   H. For people with traumatic brain injury, the Portable Neuromodulation Stimulator, or PoNS, stimulates specific nerve regions on the tongue to hopefully focus the brain on repairing the nerves that were damaged.

   I   9. human powered equipment

   I. It is a way to be developed to harness electricity from the motion of a beating heart — electricity which can then power a pacemaker. This human-generated electricity can power a range of medical devices.

   G   10. DNA legos

   J. It is a gel that instantly stops internal and external bleeding in under 10 seconds without the need to apply any pressure.

II. Translate the following sentences into Chinese.

1. The concept of precision medicine — prevention and treatment strategies that take individual variability into account — is not new; blood typing, for instance, has been used to guide blood transfusions for more than a century.

   精准医学是基于个体差异的预防与治疗策略，并不是新概念。例如，血型鉴定用于指导输血已经一个多世纪了。

2. Cancers are common diseases; in the aggregate, they are among the leading causes of death nationally and worldwide, and their incidence is increasing as the population ages.

   癌症是常见病，总体来说，癌症在美国乃至全世界都位于致死主因之列，且其发病率随人口老龄化而增长。

3. To hasten the adoption of new therapies, we will need more clinical trials with novel designs conducted in adult and pediatric patients and more reliable models for preclinical testing.

   为了加快新疗法的使用，我们需要在成人和儿童病人中进行更多设计新颖的临床试验以及建立更多可靠的临床前试验模型。

4. The initiative will encourage and support the next generation of scientists to develop creative new approaches for detecting, measuring, and analyzing a wide range of biomedical information — including molecular, genomic, cellular, clinical, behavioral, physiological, and environmental parameters.

本计划将激励并支持新生代科学家们开发创新方法，用来检测、测量并分析范围更广的生物医学信息——包括分子、基因、细胞、临床、行为、生理以及环境因素。

5. Although the precision medicine initiative will probably yield its greatest benefits years down the road, there should be some notable near-term successes.

尽管精准医学计划可能要在多年后才能产生巨大效益，但近期也会显现一些显著成果。

Ⅲ.Discuss the following topics.

1. What is precision medicine?

   Precision medicine is an emerging approach for disease treatment and prevention that takes into account individual variability in genes, environment, and lifestyle for each person.

2. What are the two main components of the Precision Medicine Initiative?

   The proposed initiative has two main components: a near-term focus on cancers and a longer-term aim to generate knowledge applicable to the whole range of health and disease.

3. Why is oncology regarded as a clear choice to enhance the impact of precision medicine?

   Cancers, as the leading causes of death nationally and worldwide, have their own genomic signature with some tumor-specific features and some features common to multiple types. Besides, inherited genetic variations contribute to cancer risk, sometimes profoundly. This new understanding of oncogenic mechanisms has begun to influence risk assessment, diagnostic categories, and therapeutic strategies, with increasing use of drugs and antibodies designed to counter the influence of specific molecular drivers.

4. What is the future of precision medicine like?

   The answer is open.

5. Are you interested in precision medicine? In what specific field are you preparing to do research?

   The answer is open.

Passage Two   First Aid in Medical Emergencies

Exercises

Ⅰ. Fill in the blanks with one proper word.

First aid, as a profession in its own right, has a history of only 120 years. It (1) <u>evolved</u> from the teachings of the Royal Humane Society and military surgeons, who saw the wisdom of training in splinting and bandaging for battlefield wounds. In 1878 two Aberdeenshire military officers, Surgeon-Major Peter Shepherd of the Royal Herbert Military Hospital, Woolwich, London, and Colonel Francis Duncan established the (2) <u>concept</u> of teaching first aid skills to civilians. This radical new enterprise, conducted (3) <u>under</u> the auspices of the newly formed

St John Ambulance Association, was a natural evolution from the body's philanthropic and ambulance transport work. Shepherd conducted the first class in the hall of the Presbyterian school in Woolwich using a comprehensive first aid curriculum that he had (4) <u>developed</u>. Within months of that first class, local Woolwich civilians used their skills when the pleasure boat Princess Alice sank in the Thames at Woolwich, killing 600 people. Within a decade, the new discipline of first aid (5) <u>spread</u> rapidly throughout the world, and by the end of the 19th century, hundreds of thousands of St John first aid certificates had been (6) <u>awarded</u> in four continents. Shepherd's pioneering classes changed the world's concept of the need for the (7) <u>provision</u> of skilled prehospital care.

From the perspective of 20th century medicine the need for first aid training seems self-evident. But first aid, (8) <u>as</u> it exists today, has a history of only about 120 years. First aid comprises a series of drills and skills which have doctrinal underpinning and which require training; the procedures are constantly revised and are (9) <u>subject</u> to ongoing medical audit. The discipline originated in 1878 from a pioneering and revolutionary experiment to teach members of the general public skills that had been developed for military stretcher bearers in the (10) <u>previous</u> decade.

II. The following are the first-aid procedures for the emergency of shock and heat stroke. Rearrange the procedures in the correct order and write the corresponding letter in the blank provided.

Shock

Shock can be life threatening. Symptoms include cold sweat, weakness, irregular breathing, chills, pale or bluish lips and fingernails, rapid weak pulse and nausea.

    4   A. Keep the victim warm (not hot) by use of blankets or clothes.

    5   B. Raise the victim's feet and legs with a pillow. (Only do this if it does not cause the victim any pain.)

    3   C. Lay the victim on his/her back, but do not move him/her if there's a back or neck injury. If the victim is unconscious, vomiting or has severe injury to the lower face or jaw, lay him/her on his/her side and be sure the victim is getting adequate air.

    1   D. Call 120 or seek medical help immediately.

    2   E. Do not give the victim anything to eat or drink.

Heat Stroke

Heat stroke can be life threatening. Symptoms can include a body temperature of 105°F or higher; dry, hot, flushed skin; rapid pulse; unconsciousness; and lack of perspiration.

    2   A. Place the victim in the shock position, lying on the back with feet up.

    1   B. Get the victim out of the heat and into a cooler place.

    5   C. Treat for shock.

    4   D. Cool the victim by fanning and applying cloth-wrapped cold packs or wet towels.

    3   E. Remove or loosen the victim's clothing.

Ⅲ.Translate the following different types of first aid into English.

1. 食物中毒   <u>food poisoning</u>   2. 癫痫   <u>epilepsy</u>
3. 窒息   <u>asphyxiation</u>   4. 扭伤   <u>sprain</u>
5. 心肌梗死   <u>myocardial infarction</u>   6. 溺水   <u>drowning</u>
7. 脑卒中   <u>stroke</u>   8. 过敏性哮喘 <u>allergic asthma</u>
9. 低血糖   <u>hypoglycemia</u>   10.骨折   <u>fracture</u>

Ⅳ.Discuss the following topics.

1. Is it necessary for medical students to acquire first-aid knowledge? Why?
   The answer is open.

2. What are the two procedures about cardiopulmonary resuscitation?
   The first procedure is getting oxygen into the blood by blowing air into the lungs. The second procedure is the application of chest pressure to compress the heart and force blood into the circulatory system.

3. Will you do it yourself if mouth-to-mouth breathing is critical to save a victim? Give your reasons.
   The answer is open.

4. What are the correct ways to treat first-degree burns and second-degree burns?
   They can be treated with a cooling lotion or cream, but more serious burns require prompt medical attention and possibly hospitalization to avoid shock and dehydration and to relieve severe pain.

Passage Three   Medical Applications for 3D Printing

Exercises

Ⅰ.Translate the following sentences into Chinese.

1. It should be cautioned that despite recent significant and exciting medical advances involving 3D printing, notable scientific and regulatory challenges remain and the most transformative applications for this technology will need time to evolve.
   <u>需要谨慎的是，尽管近年来 3D 打印取得了激动人心的、显著的医学成果，但科学性和规范管理的问题仍旧突出，该技术的转化应用尚需时日。</u>

2. Three-dimensional (3D) printing is a manufacturing method in which objects are made by fusing or depositing materials in layers to produce a 3D object.
   <u>3D 打印是一种构造物体的加工方式，利用热熔或者电铸材料逐层打印生产 3D 产品。</u>

3. The greatest advantage that 3D printers provide in medical applications is the freedom to produce custom-made medical products and equipment.
   <u>3D 打印技术赋予医疗应用最显著的优势就是自由地生产定制医疗产品和仪器。</u>

4. 3D printing has been applied in medicine since the early 2000s, when the technology was first used to make dental implants and custom prosthetics.
   <u>自 21 世纪初 3D 打印就已经开始应用于医学领域，当时，技术首先用于制作口腔植入体和定制假肢。</u>

5. 3D printing has become a useful and potentially transformative tool in a number of different fields, including medicine.

3D打印技术已经在包括医学在内的许多不同领域中成为有用且具潜力的变革性工具。

II. Here is a list of terms from the text. Analyze their meanings using the word building knowledge you have learned. Leave the space empty if the word part does not apply.

Term	Prefix	Root	Suffix	Chinese Translation
prosthetics		prosthet-	-ics	修复术
exoskeleton	exo-	skeleton		外骨骼
craniofacial		cranio-	-ial	颅面的
heterogeneous	hetero-	gen-	-ous	异质的
keratinocyte		kerato-cyte		角化细胞
fibroblast		fibro-blast		成纤维细胞